Fundamental Aspects of Men's Health

Morag Gray

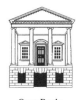

Quay Books
MA Healthcare Limited

Quay Books Division, MA Healthcare Limited, St Jude's Church, Dulwich Road, London SE24 0PB

British Library Cataloguing-in-Publication Data
A catalogue record is available for this book

Printed in the UK by Cromwell Press, Trowbridge, Wiltshire

Contents

Introduction   vii

Acknowledgements   xi

1   Men's health in context   1

2   Maintaining a healthy heart   15

3   Cancers and other diseases predominantly affecting men   41

4   Maintaining a healthy liver   77

5   Maintaining a healthy weight   88

6   Maintaining mental health   117

7   Maintaining sexual health   156

8   Conclusion   171

Index   175

Introduction

A wise man ought to realise that his health is his most valuable possession.

Hippocrates (?460–?377 BC)

Traditional epidemiological wisdom tells us that women get sicker, but men die quicker.

Hodgetts and Chamberlin (2002: 270)

For every age group, male mortality is higher than that of females, life expectancy is lower for men, men tend to use primary health services less than women, are more likely to delay help-seeking when ill and are more likely to adopt health-damaging or 'risky' behaviours, for example smoking, drinking, violence, fast driving.

Cameron and Bernardes (1998: 674)

White (2001) describes men's health as being a societal issue as opposed to a medical one, and argues that a broad approach therefore has to be taken. Lee and Owens (2002: 214) expand on this by stating, 'men's health is more than physiological functioning and more than the absence of illness; health encompasses an individual's physiological state, psychological well-being and social context.'

Faltermeyer and Pryjmachuk (2000) claim that what little information there is about men's health is concentrated solely on testicular self-examination, prostate cancer and sexual health. Rather than taking this narrow view of men's health, this book promotes a wider coverage of aspects pertinent to men's health.

Lloyd and Forrest (2001) state that there is no agreed definition of what constitutes men's health. They do however adopt Fletcher's (1997) definition in their report entitled *Boys and Young Men's Health* (2001: 5): 'conditions or diseases that are unique to men, more prevalent in men, more serious among men, for which risk factors are different for men or for which different interventions are required for men.' This definition is revised by the Men's Health Forum (2004: 5):

*A male health issue is one arising from physiological, psychological,
social, cultural or environmental factors that have a specific impact
on boys or men and/or where particular interventions are required
for boys or men in order to achieve improvements in health and well-
being at either the individual or the population level.*

These definitions have driven the material covered in this textbook. When
focusing on men's health, four elements of health promotion should be
considered: disease prevention; health education and health information; public
health promotion; and community development (Naidoo and Wills, 1998).

Most of the leading causes of death among men are the result of men's
behaviours, which then leave them more vulnerable to certain illnesses (Kimmel
and Messner, 1995). The aim of this book is to explore these behaviours and the
actions that can be taken to be proactive in improving men's health.

Box Introduction.1: Key facts about men's health

- The average male life expectancy at birth is currently 75.6 years, but
  there is variation across the country. For example, in Manchester it is
  71.0 years; in Rutland, Hart and East Dorset it is 79.5 years; and in
  Scotland it is 72.6 years.
- The average man can expect to be seriously or chronically ill for fifteen
  years of his life.
- Men who are defined as partly skilled or unskilled have a life expectancy
  of less than seventy years.
- Heart disease and stroke are, together, the biggest single cause of male
  deaths.
- Indian, Bangladeshi and Irish men have higher rates of heart disease and
  Black Caribbean, Bangladeshi and Indian men have higher rates of stroke
  than the rest of the UK male population.
- Cancer is the second most common cause of male deaths.
- Nearly 22,000 men in the UK are newly diagnosed with prostate cancer
  each year and about 9,500 die.
- The incidence of testicular cancer has increased by 15% since 1993.
- The suicide rate among men is increasing: the rate has doubled among
  fifteen to twenty-four year-old men in the past twenty-five years.
  Depression is a widespread but under-recognised problem in men.
- Sexual problems are common amongst men: almost one-fifth of men in
  their fifties experience problems maintaining or achieving an erection.
- Forty-seven per cent of men are overweight and another 21% are obese.
- Twenty-eight per cent of men smoke. The average male smoker smokes
  111 cigarettes per week.

> ⌘ Bangladeshi men are nearly twice as likely to smoke as men in the general population; smoking rates are also higher among Irish and Black Caribbean men.
>
> ⌘ Twenty-seven per cent of men drink more than the recommended limits; 36% of men aged sixteen to twenty-four years drink excessively.
>
> Source : White (2001); www.menshealthforum.org.uk

References

Cameron E, Bernardes J (1998) Gender and disadvantage in health: men's health for a change. *Sociol Health Illn* **20**(5): 673–93

Faltermeyer TS, Pryjmachuk S (2000) Men's health: concepts, criticisms and challenges. In: Kerr J (ed) *Community Health Promotion: Challenges for Practice*. London: Baillière Tindall

Fletcher R (1997) *Report on Men's Health Services*. Prepared for NSW Department of Health Men's Advisory Group, Family Action Centre. Australia: University of Newcastle

Hodgetts D, Chamberlain K (2002) The problem with men: working-class men making sense of men's health on television. *J Health Psychol* **7**(3): 269–83

Kimmel MS, Messner MA (1995) *Men's Lives*. 3rd edition. Neddham Heights, Mass: Simon & Schuster

Lee C, Owens RG (2002) Issues for a Psychology of Men's Health. *J Health Psychol* **7**(3): 209–17

Lloyd T, Forrest S (2001) *Boys' and Young Men's Health: Literature and Practice Review*. London: Health Development Agency

Men's Health Forum (2004) Getting it sorted: a policy programme for men's health. www.menshealthforum.org.uk/uploaded_files/gettingsorted2004.pdf (accessed 21 January 2005)

Naidoo J, Wills J (1998) *Practising Health Promotion: Dilemmas and Challenges*. London: Baillière Tindall

White A (2001) *Report on the Scoping Study on Men's Health*. London: Men's Health Forum

Acknowledgements

Great appreciation goes to my husband Chris for his unfailing support and encouragement. I would also like to acknowledge the early contributions of my colleagues Liz Irvine, Kevin McClure and Alison Robertson.

Chapter 1

Men's health in context

Men's health in general

> *Men's socialisation can have an impact on men's health in a range of different ways, including having little interest in health knowledge and healthy activities; becoming poor users of health services; leaving symptoms longer than necessary; and being reluctant to ask for or accept help.*
>
> Lloyd and Forrest (2001: 8)

According to Faltermeyer and Pryjmachuk (2000), there are numerous factors affecting mortality and morbidity in men:

- men generally eat less healthy diets than women
- blood pressure tends to be higher in men
- when high blood pressure is identified, men tend to ignore it
- men tend to sleep less than women
- social networks for men are smaller than for women
- the social networks that men have tend to be less intimate.

In response to the fact that men have higher rates of premature death than women, a possible explanation suggested by Hodgetts and Chamberlain (2002) is that men are stoical about their illness and reluctant to seek help. The male health website (www.menshealthforum.org.uk) suggests four possible explanations as to why men's health is so poor:

- ⌘ 'Many men are still brought up to believe that they must be strong and tough, and behave as if they are indestructible. This makes it hard for them to look after their health; in fact, it encourages risk-taking behaviours such as smoking, excessive drinking and dangerous driving. Having to be "macho" also makes it harder to ask for help from a doctor.'
- ⌘ 'Men have some built-in biological problems. The male sex hormone, testosterone, may raise the level of low density lipoproteins (LDL), the "bad" type of cholesterol that increases the risk of heart disease. Also, when men put on weight, fat tends to build up around the waist, the worst possible place in terms of developing the furred-up arteries that cause heart problems.'

⌘ 'Because men don't have periods, they lack a mechanism that regularly and naturally makes them feel aware of, and in touch with, their bodies. What's more, men's reproductive systems don't require them to maintain any regular contact with health care services. They don't eed to see a doctor to obtain contraception and, of course, they don't get pregnant.'

⌘ 'Health services haven't done much to encourage men to look after their health. Most GP's surgeries are still only open at times when men are likely to be at work, for example, and often don't feel like male-friendly places. There's also been chronic under-investment in research into male-specific problems, especially prostate disease.'

In White's (2001a) work on the scoping of men's health, he found four areas emerging from his analysis: men's access to health services; men's lack of awareness of their health needs; men's seeming inability to express emotions; and men's lack of social networks. These themes will form the basis for the next section of this chapter.

Men's lack of awareness of their health needs

A common finding from the literature on men's health is the explanation that men's lack of awareness of their health needs is due to how they are socialised into their male role. This in effect leaves them vulnerable to certain illnesses (Lloyd and Forrest, 2001). Men are brought up to believe that in order to portray their maleness or masculinity, they should behave in certain ways. From a societal perspective, in general, men are seen to be combative, competitive, independent and naturally strong (Davidson and Lloyd, 2001; Lee and Owens, 2002). Men tend to see illness as something that happens to others and that sickness is a sign of weakness. The belief that they are naturally strong and in control leads to the belief that they are somehow resistant to disease and should be unresponsive to pain and unconcerned with minor symptoms (Lloyd and Forrest, 2001; White, 2001a; Lee and Owens, 2002). This leads men to be stoical, silent and to 'keep a stiff upper lip' (Pringle, undated).

It is generally thought that this socialisation process directly impacts on how men perceive and know their bodies. Auon *et al* (2002) carried out research aimed at assessing the effectiveness of a health intervention for men. They used focus-group interviews with a sample of 525 men in their workplace setting. One of their findings was that men don't take the same level of interest in their health that women do in theirs, with the consequence, as one of their participants stated, that men tend to 'self-destruct.' The researchers also found that men tended to view potentially serious symptoms as signs of growing old, which reflects a general lack of health-related knowledge. Lloyd and Forrest (2001) assert that not only do men have a tendency to ignore serious symptoms, but they also have a tendency to play them down when they do eventually seek help, which in turn can cause the doctor to underestimate their severity.

It is known that men do not have the same level of awareness of the functioning of their bodies as women. One consequence is that men may not appreciate bodily changes as quickly as women do, which builds in a delay that could have serious implications with regard to the course of the disease (White 2001a). This is reinforced by Lantz *et al* (2001) who report that women are much likelier than men to identify and report subtle symptoms. Men tend to wait until their symptoms are more concrete, by which time the disease may be more advanced and treatment less effective.

White (2001b: 18) expresses what Lantz *et al* (2001) refer to as macho social conditioning: 'part of the problem lies in the relationship men have with their bodies. A man's body is central to masculinity and of ensuring that the man's self-image is in keeping with the expectations of society. Masculinity contains a strong element of control and most men take it for granted that the body's workings will be mastered... Culturally, women's bodies are seen as open, both in relation to sexual penetration and through giving birth or menstruating; men's bodies are seen as closed, strong and invincible, as is evident from the risk-taking men engage in. Men are also conditioned to see their bodies as the boundary between the unknown inside (which includes their emotions and sexual inclinations) and the potentially invasive outside... It's only when the body starts to go wrong that the man begins to realise how vulnerable his body actually is.'

White (2001a: 11) suggests that the following factors be considered to improve men's awareness of their health needs:

- ⌘ 'Work with mothers and fathers from antenatal care onwards regarding what are normal developmental processes for boys and that they generally need more affection than girls, not less.'
- ⌘ 'Parents need guidance on the specific difficulties boys have with understanding their health.'
- ⌘ 'Enhancing the role of Sure Start initiative to help give boys in primary school an understanding of their health, especially those from areas of deprivation.'
- ⌘ 'Work with the Healthy Schools initiative to develop within boys:
  - ❖ A clearer understanding of the male body and the possible health risks they face.
  - ❖ Healthy models of maleness that boys and men can follow — the appropriate "heroes".
  - ❖ An appreciation of the benefits of exercise and healthy diets.'
- ⌘ 'School holiday clubs need to incorporate a health focus.'
- ⌘ 'The closer integration between local health services and schools to enable health professionals to work alongside teachers to deliver the agenda within schools.'

⌘ 'The inclusion of school boys' health within the local health strategy as outlined in local Health Improvement Plans (HimPs) and Health Action Zones (HAZs)...'

⌘ 'Health strategies for men in the local community should include plans to increase awareness of men of all ages to the benefits of exercise in terms of fitness and health but also in terms of companionship.'

Lantz *et al* (2001) add that earlier socialisation of boys should include the idea that seeking health advice is a positive and not a negative action, since being healthy will enhance their self-image. It is known that men make use of the internet to access health information (Lantz *et al*, 2001; White, 2001a). Baker (2001) notes that confidential and anonymous forms of help seem most popular with men as do 'pub-clinics', which remain a rarity.

Men's access to health services

In the Cameron and Bernardes (1998) survey of 565 men with prostatitis and benign enlarged prostates, it was discovered that men tend to view health and health-related activity as the province of the female. This finding is reinforced by Lantz *et al* (2001) and O'Leary (2001) who state that men adopt a passive role towards their health and have a tendency to rely on their family and friends to seek help. It could be argued that this behaviour provides men with a social sanction to seek help in that they have been pushed to see their GP at the insistence of others.

White (2001a) states that up until the age of sixteen, boys and girls attend their GP equally as their mother takes them, but that, after that age, men have a great reluctance to attend. It is suggested that when men do attend their GP, which may be between two and four times a year, it is for treatment as opposed to any kind of preventative health care. The delay in seeking treatment can contribute to morbidity and even premature mortality.

One of the key factors affecting prognosis following a myocardial infarction (heart attack) is the time taken to seek treatment. Delay in seeking treatment has a direct effect on morbidity and mortality. The administration of thrombolytic agents must take place soon after the onset of symptoms to minimise cell death and reduce both morbidity and mortality (Caldwell and Miaskowski, 2002). There have been a number of research studies that have investigated why men delay in seeking treatment when they experience chest pains.

White and Johnson (2000) carried out a grounded theory study to investigate why men delayed in seeking help. They undertook participant observation of twenty-five men who had been admitted with acute chest pain, followed by in-depth interviews of ten of these men following discharge. They found that delay was due to one of two processes: rationalisation and denial. Rationalisation involved the men explaining that their pain was due to indigestion, anaemia or normal ageing — they therefore put up with the symptoms. Denial resulted from the men realising that there was potential for the pains to have serious causes, which increased their feelings of vulnerability — and, in turn, led them to use denial as a coping mechanism. White and Johnson (2000) reported that the men did not rate themselves as being at risk in the first place, and most were surprised to hear that they had had a myocardial infarction.

Richards *et al* (2002) used qualitative interviews with a purposive sample of thirty men and thirty women from the age group forty-five to sixty-four years who had experienced chest pain. The participants were from two economically contrasting areas of Glasgow, Scotland, UK. The aim of the research was to ascertain whether the responses to chest pain varied with socioeconomic status or sex. The researchers found that individuals from the more deprived areas felt more vulnerable to coronary heart disease because of a strong family history, and were likely to have witnessed angina and deaths from coronary heart disease in young relatives. They were also more likely to report negative experiences with health care; hold lower expectations of health care; and the perception that they were to blame for their condition and would be chastised by their GP.

Richards *et al* (2002) suggest that the socially deprived barriers in seeking help are fear, denial, low expectations, and diagnostic confusion. They found that individuals from more affluent areas were more likely to deny a family history of coronary heart disease and distance themselves from any risk of it by using the third person when discussing it at interview. The more affluent individuals reported greater formal knowledge and more extensive sharing of knowledge with their GP. Overall, there were three reasons why individuals from more socially deprived areas didn't seek help for their chest pain. First, they normalised their pain; second, they were unable to distinguish their chest pain from other types of pain, such as chest infection or indigestion; and, third, since they were likely to have other health problems as well as their chest pain, they were concerned that they may be overusing medical services.

From White's research (2001a), the following list of reasons was given as a set of indicators to explain why men are generally reluctant to go to their GP:

⌘ A lack of understanding of the processes of making appointments and negotiating with female receptionists.

⌘ Inappropriate opening times, which tend to coincide with work commitments.

⌘ An unwillingness to wait for appointments.

⌘ A feeling that the service is primarily for women and children, making sitting in the waiting room uncomfortable for them.

⌘ Even the name 'health centre' has been identified as problematic.

⌘ The negative response many men feel they get when presenting with difficulties that are not quickly dealt with.

⌘ A lack of trust in the system, mainly around the issue of confidentiality, especially within the gay community and disclosure of HIV status.

⌘ Great fears relating to shame if their concerns are judged to be of little consequence, or having to admit to another person that you may have a problem, and one that you can't solve.

⌘ Lacking the vocabulary they feel they need to discuss issues of a sensitive nature, with the result that it is easier to go to the doctor with a non-embarrassing physical illness then when depressed or faced with the symptoms of, say, colorectal cancer or erectile dysfunction.

Pringle (undated) shares his research findings regarding men's views of visiting their GP. He found, in common with other research, that men used their GP only as a last resort and that when they did visit they found the waiting rooms unfriendly, the receptionists difficult and judgmental, and their GP having limited time to spend with them and being patronising towards them. When men do see their GP, it is usually with symptoms that keep their male image intact (Davidson and Lloyd, 2001). In Lantz *et al*'s (2001) study, men reported that the major reason for going to their GP was the need for a physical examination for employment or insurance purposes.

Evidently, when men do visit their GPs, it tends to be related to symptoms of an illness rather than engaging in health-promotion activities. Again, women seem to play a dominant role here too. Leishman and Dalziel (2003) explain that divorced and single men are less likely to have their cholesterol levels and blood pressure checked routinely than are married men. The latter group was more likely to have been 'bossed' by their wives into attending for routine check-ups. According to Davidson and Lloyd (2001), living with a female partner appears to improve men's health.

Men who live alone are much more likely to smoke, drink alcohol excessively, and have an unhealthy diet. However, even with the acknowledgement of the women's role, men are much less likely to adopt preventative health behaviours then women (Lee and Owens, 2002). Since health behaviours are directly related to one's health and longevity, this contributes to morbidity and mortality in men (Courtney, 2000; Courtenay *et al*, 2002).

Auon *et al* (2002) report that men are generally less motivated to change their health behaviours: younger men believe it's too early and older men believe it's too late. According to Auon *et al* (2002), the barriers to change include the difficulty of changing established routines; a lack of personal discipline; and scepticism about apparently contradictory medical advice.

Barton (2000) provides some useful guidelines for the development of health promotion services for men:

- ⌘ 'Anonymity and privacy: protecting men from "losing face" (the majority of callers to health helplines are men).'
- ⌘ 'Work-based services are well used by men; the worker role allows expression of health needs that affect their job.'
- ⌘ 'Concrete, practical services such as vasectomy clinics are good entry points to other health facilities.'
- ⌘ 'Reaching men when they are in crisis is effective.'
- ⌘ 'Presenting issues in terms of fitness and good health paradoxically allows men to admit to ill health.'
- ⌘ 'Targeting men helps to build a picture of their needs; targeting men in pubs, clubs and sport centres is necessary because of their reluctance to attend traditional health settings.'
- ⌘ 'Promoting the service through local networks, local newspapers, local workplaces, other health service entry gates, pubs, clubs, sports centres and so on.'

Barton (2000) adds pertinent advice for nurses involved in health-promotion initiatives aimed at men: make sure the environment is conducive and safe for men; advertise the service/event extensively; and hold the event in the evening with no appointment needed so men can drop in as best suits them. This advice is endorsed by Deville-Almond (2001), Lloyd and Forrest (2001) and Parish (2001).

Men's seeming inability to express emotions

Men are less likely than women to seek help for emotional problems; when they do, they are less likely to receive appropriate treatment (Lee and Owens, 2002). From White's (2001a: 13) work, the following solutions were suggested to help boys and men understand their emotions better:

- ⌘ 'Work with the Healthy Schools initiative to develop within boys an emotional literacy to enable them to be able to recognise and articulate their worries.'
- ⌘ 'Recognition of the differing forms of depression within men, and how different cultures portray mental health difficulties.'
- ⌘ 'Need to de-stigmatise depression within society to allow men to come forward and seek help.'
- ⌘ 'Recognition of the increasing stress that men are under at work.'
- ⌘ 'Recognition that the models of maleness that are prevalent at the moment militate against rather than for men's mental health.'

Men's lack of social networks

A social network can be described as a set of relationships that an individual has with others such as friends, family and neighbours. Nutbeam (1998: 19) defines a social network as 'social relations and links between individuals which may provide access to or mobilization of social support for health.' He goes on to state that high unemployment, re-housing schemes and rapid urbanization can all lead to the dissolution of social networks.

It is through social networks that there is expression of positive regard; acknowledgement of others' feelings and beliefs; encouragement of open expression of feelings and beliefs; and the offer of advice and information. Women tend to have a much stronger social network of friends and supportive systems than do men (Matthews *et al*, 1999; White, 2001b).

The manner by which men and women use their social networks differs. Women's friendships focus on intimacy and disclosure, whilst men's emphasise sociability and have a task-orientation. Men tend to maintain a close intimate relationship with only a very few people and primarily their spouse (Bansal *et al*, 2000). Bansal *et al* (2000) report that individuals who have greater social support tend to experience less psychological distress during stressful events.

Antonucci *et al* (2003) note that males who were less educated had better health when they had larger social networks, and worse health when they had small social networks. It is known that, generally, individuals in the lower socioeconomic groups are less healthy than those in the higher socioeconomic groups. Martikainen *et al* (2003) found that being a smoker and not taking exercise was related to having an unhealthy diet. Of those men who had very unhealthy diets, more than 40% were from the lower socioeconomic groups.

Risk-taking behaviour

Adolescence is generally described as a transitional phase of development that begins at the onset of puberty and continues into early adulthood.

Spear and Kulbok (2001: 83)

Risk-taking involves a range of behaviours often associated with alcohol consumption, including taking drugs they would not have otherwise; having unprotected sex; being involved in an argument or fight; and driving under the influence of alcohol.

Purser (2001)

Risk-taking is defined by Gullone and Moore (2000: 393) as 'participation in behaviour which involves potential negative consequences (or loss) balanced in some way by perceived positive consequences (or gain).' Risk-taking behaviour is predominantly associated with adolescents and young men. Lloyd and Forrest (2001) argue that taking risks is related to how masculinity is socially constructed and identify four types of risk:

1. those that are socially sanctioned
2. those that involve thrill seeking
3. those that reflect rebellious risk
4. those that are reckless and anti-social

Adolescence is a transitional phase of life and is strongly associated with the development of risk-taking in activities such as smoking, drinking alcohol, drug abuse and sexual health (Kiddy, 2002). In their literature review on boy's and men's health, Lloyd and Forrest (2001: 2) cite Calman's (1994) more developed views on adolescence as 'the transitional phase between childhood and adulthood, characterised by experimentation and rapid change. It is a key time for learning, mainly by exploration of new ideas and behaviours, for consolidating health-related values, attitudes and lifestyles, and for making decisions about various behaviours which have important consequences for future health. The purpose of adolescent healthcare is to support this process and to enable young people to become healthy and competent adults.'

By taking physical risks, individuals demonstrate their competence and courage (Lee and Owens, 2002). Courtenay (2000) expands on this in relation to men taking health risks, such as refusing to take sick leave; insisting that they need little sleep in order to function; and boasting that drinking alcohol does not impair their driving ability. Taking these health risks, states Courtenay (2000), validates men as the 'stronger sex'.

According to Greene *et al* (2000), there are three theories as to why adolescents and young men engage in risk behaviours. One theory involving a personality characteristic seeks to explain why some individuals engage in risky behaviours more than others. It is associated with the trait of sensation-seeking, which is reported to peak during adolescence. The sensation-seeking trait, according to Ulleberg (2002), indicates a need to experience novelty, excitement and danger. It is associated with cocaine use, lax attitudes about sexual behaviour, risky driving behaviour, and alcohol use (Greene, 2000). The second theory is based on risk-taking being a learned behaviour and, as such, a form of social deviance. The third theory explains risk-taking as being due to developmental immaturity or lack of experience, which may lead to errors in judgement (Greene *et al*, 2000). Related to the developmental theory, Alcohol Concern (2004: 1) cites Thom and Francome's (2001) work, which identified common developmental predictors that are shared with a number of risk-taking activities. These predictors include:

- 'disrupted family background'
- 'poor parental supervision and communication'
- 'problems at school'
- 'poor social skills'
- 'physical or sexual abuse in childhood'
- 'having a risk-seeking personality'
- 'having a history of age-inappropriate behaviour'

For males, the following factors in particular have been found to be associated with alcohol use and other risky behaviours:

- ⌘ 'Involvement with "delinquent" groups or having "delinquent" siblings.'
- ⌘ 'Feeling alienated.'
- ⌘ 'Males seem to be under more pressure to drink.'
- ⌘ 'Males face greater expectations that alcohol will be accompanied by increased aggression and fighting.'
- ⌘ 'Males are under pressure to adopt a "macho" image in relation to alcohol use.'
- ⌘ 'Alcohol use is associated with, and is frequently used as an excuse for, bad behaviour, including aggression and offending.'

A number of structural and cultural factors also come into play when looking at alcohol and risk. These include:

- 'underage drinking'
- 'drinking venues'
- 'cultural norms and values regarding drinking and drinking behaviour.'

Road traffic accidents

If you drink, don't drive. Don't even putt.

Dean Martin

Road traffic accidents are the single greatest cause of death among young people. 'Risk-taking behaviour combined with lack of experience and alcohol and to a lesser extent, drugs, are significant factors in accident causation for this age group.' (Davidson and Lloyd, 2001: 27). Younger drivers are more likely to drive too fast, follow too closely, and overtake dangerously compared with other drivers (Ulleberg, 2002). Recent figures also show that young male drivers and riders are twice as likely to fail a breath test than other road users (Alcohol Concern, 2004). Young men between sixteen and twenty-four are the heaviest-drinking section of the UK population.

How alcohol contributes to accidents

According to Alcohol Concern (2003: 2), 'The present drink-driving limit is 80mg of alcohol to 100ml of blood but changes to driving performance can occur at lower and higher levels.' They continue:

⌘ 'At 20–50mg blood alcohol concentration (BAC) (1.5–3 units for men and 0.5–2 units for women), the ability to see or locate moving lights correctly is diminished, as is the ability to judge distances. The tendency to take risks is increased.'

⌘ 'At 50–80mg alcohol/100ml blood (3–5 units for men, 2–3 for women), the ability to judge distances is reduced, so is the adaptability of the eyes to changing light conditions, and sensitivity to red lights is also impaired. Reactions are slower and concentration span is shorter. By the time the legal limit is reached, drinkers are 5 times more likely to have a driving accident than before they starting drinking.'

⌘ 'At 80–120mg alcohol/100ml blood (5–8 units for men, 3–5 for women), euphoria sets in and with it an over-estimation of one's abilities, leading to reckless driving. The driver will begin to suffer impairment of peripheral vision (resulting in accidents due to hitting vehicles in passing), impairment of perception of obstacles and of ability to assess dimension. At 120mg alcohol/100ml blood, the driver is 10 times as likely to have an accident.'

White (2001a) points out that accidents and risk-taking are closely linked to young people's feelings of invulnerability and their desire to be seen as being strong and able. He also stresses that legislation, such as the compulsory wearing of seat belts and motorcycle helmets, has been required to reduce accident rates.

Young drivers have a tendency to estimate, inaccurately, their driving skills as being superior to those of their peers and older drivers, and to judge that they have a much lower risk of being involved in a crash or being caught for speeding than others. As young men make the transition into adulthood, the majority outgrow risky driving behaviours (Begg and Langley, 2001).

Box 1.1: Strategies to minimise dangers of drinking

- ⌘ Know the legal limits and stick to them. (The current legal limit for driving is 80mg of alcohol per 100ml of blood, but this is under review by the Government in relation to adopting the legal limit in the rest of Europe, which is 50mg of alcohol per 100ml of blood.)
- ⌘ Eat and drink something 'soft' before going out, since alcohol is absorbed fastest when the stomach is empty.
- ⌘ Drink water in between alcoholic drinks.
- ⌘ When in a group, nominate if possible a non-drinking person to 'look after' the others.
- ⌘ Use taxis rather than walking, and drink in known safe places.
- ⌘ Do not attempt to drink and drive.

Source: UK Youth (2003);
http://www.youthinformation.com/infopage.asp?snID=825
(last accessed January 2005)

References

Alcohol Concern (2004) Alcohol and men factsheet. http://www.alcoholconcern.org. uk/servlets/doc/686 (last accessed February 2005)

Alcohol Concern (2003) Factsheet 9: alcohol and accidents. http://www. alcoholconcern.org.uk/servlets/doc/250 (last accessed February 2005)

Antonucci TC, Ajrouch KJ, Janevic MR (2003) The effect of social relations with children on the education-health link in men and women aged 40 and over. *Soc Sci Med* **56**: 949–60

Auon S, Donovan RJ, Johnson L, Egger G (2002) Preventative care in the context of men's health. *J Health Psychol* **7**(3): 243–52

Baker P (2001) The state we're in: an overview of men's health. Tackling the inequalities. Report of a one-day multidisciplinary conference. http://www. menshealthforum.org.uk/uploaded_files/mhjstate.pdf (last accessed February 2005)

Bansal A, Monnier J, Hobfoll SE, Stone B (2000) Comparing men's and women's loss of perceived social and work resources following psychological distress. *J Soc Pers Relat* **17**(2): 265–81

Barton A (2000) Men's health: a cause for concern. *Nurs Stand* **15**(10): 47–52

Begg D, Langley J (2001) Changes in risky driving behaviour from age 21 to 26 years. *J Safety Res* **32**(4): 491–9

Caldwell MA, Miaskowski C (2002) Mass media interventions to reduce help-seeking delay in people with symptoms of acute myocardial infarction: time for a new approach. *Patient Educ Couns* **46**: 1–9

Calman K (1994) *On the State of the Public Health*. London: HMSO

Cameron E, Bernardes J (1998) Gender and disadvantage in health: men's health for a change. *Sociol Health Illn* **20**(5): 673–93

Courtenay WH, McCreary DR, Merighi JR (2002) Gender and ethnic differences in health beliefs and behaviours. *J Health Psychol* **7**(3): 219–31

Courtney WH (2000) Constructions of masculinity and their influence on men's well-being: a theory of gender and health. *Soc Sci Med* **50**: 1385–1401

Davidson N, Lloyd T, eds (2001) *Promoting Men's Health: A Guide for Practitioners*. Edinburgh: Baillière Tindall

Deville-Almond J (2001) Primary care: what can we do? Tackling the inequalities. Report of a one-day multidisciplinary conference. http://www.menshealthforum. org.uk/userpage1.cfm?item_id=756 (last accessed February 2005)

Faltermeyer TS, Pryjmachuk S (2000) Men's health: concepts, criticisms and challenges. In: Kerr J (ed) *Community Health Promotion: Challenges for Practice*. London: Baillière Tindall

Fletcher R (1997) *Report on Men's Health Services*. Prepared for NSW Department of Health Men's Advisory Group. Family Action Centre. Australia: University of Newcastle

Greene K, Kramar M, Walters LH, Rubin DL, Hale J, Hale L (2000) Targeting adolescent risk-taking behaviours: the contribution of egocentrism and sensation-seeking. *J Adolesc* **23**: 439–61

Gullone E, Moore S (2000) Adolescent risk-taking and the five-factor model or personality. *J Adolesc* **23**: 393–407

Hodgetts D, Chamberlain K (2002) The problem with men: working-class men making sense of men's health on television. *J Health Psychol* **7**(3): 269–83

Kiddy M (2001) Teenage pregnancy: whose problem? *Nurs Times* **98**(4): 36–7

Lantz JM, Fullerton JT, Harshburger RJ, Sadler GR (2001) Promoting screening and early detection of cancer in men. *Nurs Health Sci* **3**: 189–96

Lee C, Owens RG (2002) Issues for a psychology of men's health. *J Health Psychol* **7**(3): 209–17

Leishman J, Dalziel A (2003) Taking action to improve the health of Scottish men. *Men's Health Journal* **2**(2): 90–3

Lloyd T, Forrest S (2001) Boys' and young men's health: literature and practice review. London: Health Development Agency

Martikainen P, Brunner E, Marmot M (2003) Socioeconomic differences in dietary patterns among middle-aged men and women. *Soc Sci Med* **56**: 1397–1410

Matthews S, Stansfield S, Power C (1999) Social support at age 33: the influence of gender, employment status and social class. *Soc Sci Med* **49**: 133–42

Men's Health Forum (2004) Getting it Sorted: a Policy Programme for Men's Health. Men's Health Forum. http://www.menshealthforum.org.uk/uploaded_files/ gettingsorted2004.pdf (last accessed January 2005)

Nutbeam D (1998) *Health Promotion Glossary*. Geneva: WHO

O'Leary S (2001) Getting men to see the doctor. Tackling the inequalities. Report of a one-day multidisciplinary conference. http://www.menshealthforum.org.uk/userpage1.cfm?item_id=277 (last accessed February 2005)

Parish P (2001) Tackling men's health inequalities: what can the government do? Tackling the inequalities. Report of a one-day multidisciplinary conference. http://www.menshealthforum.org.uk/userpage1.cfm?item_id=756 (last accessed February 2005)

Pringle A (undated) Developing accessible health services for men. http://www.menshealthforum.org.uk/userpage1.cfm?item_id=239 (last accessed January 2005)

Purser B, Orford J, Johnson M (2001) *Drinking in Second and Subsequent Black and Asian Communities in the English Midlands.* London: Alcohol Concern

Richards HM, Reid ME, Watt GCM (2002) Socioeconomic variations in responses to chest pain: qualitative study. *BMJ* **324**: 1308–11

Spear HJ, Kulbok PA (2001) Adolescent health behaviors and related factors: a review. *Public Health Nurs* **18**(2): 82–93

Thom B, Francome C (2001) Men at risk: risk taking, substance use and gender. London: Middlesex University

Ulleberg P (2002) Personality subtypes of young drivers. Relationship to risk-taking preferences, accident involvement, and response to a traffic safety campaign. *Transport Res* **4**: 279–97

UK Youth (2003) *Young Men and Alcohol: a Good Practice Guide to Peer Education.* London: UK Youth

White A (2001a) Report on the Scoping Study on Men's Health. Leeds: Leeds Metropolitan University

White A (2001b) How men respond to illness. *Men's Health J* **1**(1): 18–19

White AK, Johnson M (2000) Men making sense of their chest pain — niggles, doubts and denials. *J Clin Nurs* **9**: 534–41

Chapter 2

Maintaining a healthy heart

Cardiovascular disease (CVD) is the main cause of death in the UK, accounting for just under 238,000 deaths a year: 39% of all deaths.

British Heart Foundation [BHF] (2004)

Coronary heart disease is largely preventable.

Wanless (2002: 22)

A staggering 2.7 million people are estimated to be living with coronary heart disease in the UK — a number that is rising year on year.

BHF (2004)

Coronary heart disease (CHD)

Coronary heart disease (CHD) is defined by Wallis *et al* (2000: 671) as 'a fatal or non-fatal myocardial infarction plus incident angina. Cardiovascular disease is defined as coronary heart disease but also including stroke, peripheral vascular disease and heart failure.' Primatesta (1998) explains that there is a hierarchy of diseases making up cardiovascular diseases and these are, from greatest severity to least, myocardial infarction (heart attack) or stroke; angina; high blood pressure or diabetes; murmur or irregular heart rhythm or other heart trouble. CHD alone is responsible for around 17,000 deaths every year in Scotland, which has one of the highest CHD mortality rates in the Western world (Inchley *et al*, 2001).

Scotland's health record remains poor. Some £1.25 billion spent in 1996–97 on incapacity and invalidity benefit in Scotland to people not well enough to work is one measure of the extent of ill health. The life expectancy at birth for both sexes in Scotland in 1994 was lower than that in many other industrialised countries. Among these countries, Scotland has the highest mortality rate from CHD for men and the second highest for women. The prevalence of CHD among men aged fifty-five to sixty-four years in Scotland is almost one-in-six compared with one-in-ten in England in the same age group (Working Together for a Healthier Scotland, 1998).

Tod *et al* (2001) found that there were both regional and socioeconomic differences in the incidence of CHD. The death rates from CHD in Barnsley, Rotherham and Doncaster are among the highest in England and Wales. The premature death rate from CHD for men living in Scotland is 50% higher than that in men living in East Anglia (DoH, 1999). Socioeconomic deprivation is known to have a profound effect on the risk of having a myocardial infarction. Most deprived members of society under sixty-five years of age have double the risk of having a myocardial infarction and death before reaching hospital, and 20% are more likely to die within the first month following myocardial infarction (Macintyre *et al*, 2001).

Indian, Pakistani and particularly Bangladeshi men are about twice as likely to experience CHD than men in the general population (BHF, 2002). Chinese and Black-Caribbean men have a lower incidence of CHD than those in the general population. Bangladeshi men eat more red meat and fried foods and less fruit than men in other ethnic groups. However, Indian men are less likely to eat red meat and fried foods. Chinese men have the highest fruit and vegetable consumption of all the ethnic groups. The lowest level of vegetable consumption is in the Pakistani community (DoH, 1999).

As with other diseases, it is generally accepted that socioeconomic factors influence the overall rates of CHD events (Macintyre *et al*, 2001):

> *The adult social status influences both the socioeconomic*
> *environment (unfavourable micro and macro economic aspects,*
> *insufficient healthcare utilisation, poor social networks and*
> *working conditions) and the individual emotional reactions (lack*
> *of self-esteem and coping mechanisms, poor sense of coherence,*
> *hopelessness, depression, hostility and anger). These may in turn be*
> *reflected in unhealthy lifestyle patterns (smoking, poor dietary habits,*
> *lack of physical activity and obesity) and thus unfavourably influence*
> *the pathogenesis of cardiovascular diseases.*

Wood *et al* (1998: 1449)

As a result, there are unequal effects of CHD. Unskilled men, for example, have a death rate that is three times higher than that for professional men, and these differences have more than doubled in the past twenty years (DoH, 2000).

One of the major risk factors associated with CHD is smoking. It is important to note that whilst the proportion of young people who start to smoke is similar across the social classes, by the time they are in their thirties, 50% of individuals who are socioeconomically 'better off' have stopped smoking — whereas 75% of those in lower income groups continue. The risk of developing CHD in the future is particularly high if individuals start smoking before the age of fifteen years (Wood *et al*, 1998). According to DoH (1999) 'this is powerful evidence of how the cycle of social disadvantage contributes directly to the risk of premature death, avoidable illness and disability. About one third of smokers are concentrated in the bottom 10% of earners in this country.' In Scotland, smoking is said to account for more than 13,000 deaths every year and costs the NHS £140 million in treating smoking-related diseases (Hunt *et al*, 2000).

Box 2.1: Key facts about coronary heart disease (CHD)

⌘ Coronary heart disease (CHD) is largely preventable — physical inactivity, obesity, smoking and diabetes are major risk factors.

⌘ Age-standardised death rates for CHD show that the UK, particularly cotland and Northern Ireland, has one of the highest rates compared with most other industrialised countries.

⌘ CHD affects more than 1.4 million people in the UK and about 268,000 have a heart attack each year, which equates to one every two minutes.

⌘ CHD is the leading cause of death in the West.

⌘ In the UK, one in four men die from CHD.

⌘ Nearly all deaths from CHD are due to myocardial infarctions.

⌘ Twenty-two per cent of premature deaths in men are due to cardiovascular disease.

⌘ The premature death rate for CHD in men living in Scotland is almost 50% higher than for men in the south-west of England.

⌘ South Asian (Indian, Bangladeshi, Pakistani and Sri Lankan) men living in the UK have a 46% higher premature death rate from CHD than average.

⌘ Premature death rate from CHD in male manual workers is 58% higher than in male non-manual workers.

⌘ Premature death rate from stroke is 36% higher in manual workers than in non-manual workers.

⌘ The death rate for non-manual workers is falling faster than that for manual workers.

⌘ A working-age man is more than twice as likely to die from CHD in the UK than in Italy.

⌘ It is estimated that there are about 174,000 new cases of angina in men each year.

⌘ It is estimated that there are 33,000 new cases of heart failure in men each year.

⌘ The incidence of heart attack increases with age and is more common in men than in women.

⌘ CHD costs the UK economy a total of £7,055 million per year.

Sources: Scottish Office Department of Health (1998); Primatesta (1998);
Richardson (2000); British Nutrition Foundation [BNF] (2004);
WHO (2001); BHF (2002, 2004).

Risk factors

There are five major risk factors for developing CHD (*Table 2.1*):

Table 2.1: Five major risk factors for developing CHD				
Risk factor	**US estimates**	**UK estimates**		
		Men	Women	All
Blood cholesterol >5.2mmol/l	43%	45%	47%	46%
Physical activity <twelve 20–min occasions of vigorous activity in the past 4 weeks	35%	36%	38%	37%
Blood pressure >149/90mmHg	25%	14%	12%	13%
Smoking	22%	20%	17%	19%
Obesity (BMI >=30)	17%	5%	6%	6%

Source: BHF (2002)

Each risk factor will now be discussed in some detail.

Diet

Having an unhealthy diet is also a cause of CHD. Indeed, some 30% of deaths from CHD are said to be attributable to unhealthy diets and 45% of deaths in men from CHD are attributable to raised blood cholesterol levels (over 5.2mmol/l). The mean blood cholesterol level for men in England is 5.5 mmol/l and some 66% have levels exceeding 5 mmol/l. A 10% reduction in blood cholesterol lowers the risk of developing CHD by 50% at the age of 40% and 20% at the age of 70. A poor diet is a fact of life for many poorer families (DoH, 1999). Eating oily fish also contributes to a reduction in risk of developing CHD as oily fish contains polyunsaturated fatty acids which reduce blood viscosity and thereby inhibit clot formation (BNF, 2001).

The UK government's Committee on the Medical Aspects of Food and Nutrition Policy (COMA) made recommendations in 1994, which specified a number of measures to improve our diet. These measures included reducing our saturated fat and salt intake and increasing our carbohydrate, fruit and vegetable consumption. It is now commonly quoted that we should all eat at least five portions of fruit and vegetables every day. However, the National

Diet and Nutrition survey found that whilst the eating of fresh fruit has increased fourfold since the 1940s, the intake of fresh vegetables has decreased. Moreover, the survey indicated that only 16% of boys in the two-to-fifteen years age group eat fruit more than once a day. There are also regional differences in the UK: people in Scotland, Ireland and the north of England consume fewer fruits and vegetables than their counterparts in the south of England. The BNF (2002) stated that people in London consumed almost twice as many fruits and vegetables as those in Northern Ireland.

According to the BHF (2004), 88% of men consume too much saturated fat and 85% consume too much salt. In terms of fat and saturated-fat intake, there are no variations between social groups. However, there are considerable differences when it comes to fruits and vegetables, with those in higher socioeconomic groups eating more than those in lower socioeconomic groups. *Table 2.2 (pp. 20–21)*suggests food choices that should be made to lower saturated fats within one's diet.

Indian, Pakistani and particularly Bangladeshi men are about twice as likely to experience CHD than men in the general population. Chinese and Black Caribbean men have a lower incidence of CHD than those in the general population. Indian, Pakistani and particularly Bangladeshi men are about twice as likely to experience CHD than men in the general population (BHF, 2002). Bangladeshi men eat more red meat and fried foods, and less fruit, than men in other ethnic groups. However, Indian men are less likely to eat red meat and are less likely to eat fried foods. Chinese men have the highest fruit and vegetable consumption compared with men from other ethnic groups. The lowest level of vegetable consumption is amongst the Pakistani community (DoH, 1999).

Exercise

Regular aerobic exercise helps reduce the risk of developing CHD, as it prevents or slows the laying down of atherosclerotic plaque in blood vessels (Woolf-May *et al*, 1999). Haapanen *et al* (1997) suggest that physical activity has a preventative effect not only on CHD, but also on hypertension and diabetes. The BNF (2002) estimates that 38% of deaths from CHD are due to a lack of exercise. The recommendation is for adults to exercise aerobically for at least 30 minutes, five days per week. Apparently, only 37% of men in the UK meet this recommendation. It is also recommended that children (five to eighteen years) undertake some form of moderate exercise for at least one hour per day. In England, it is reported that 55% of boys meet this target. Six out of ten men are not physically active enough to benefit their health (DoH, 1999).

Table 2.2: Food choices for a healthy lipid lowering diet

	Recommended foods (low in fat and/or high in fibre)	Foods for use in moderation (contain unsaturated fats or smaller quantities of saturated fats)	Foods only for exceptional use (contain large proportions of saturated fats and/or cholesterol, or sugar and therefore should be avoided wherever possible)
Cereals	Wholegrain bread, wholegrain breakfast cereals, porridge, cereals, whole grain pasta and rice, crispbread	White pasta and rice	
Dairy products	Skimmed milk, very low fat cheeses, e.g. cottage cheese, fat-free fromage frais or quark, fat-free yoghurt, egg white, egg substitutes	Semi-skimmed milk, fat-reduced and lower fat cheeses eg. Camembert, Edam, feta, ricotta, low-fat yoghurt. Two whole eggs per week	Whole milk, condensed milk, cream, imitation milk, full-fat cheeses e.g. Brie, Gouda, full-fat yoghurt
Soups	Consommés, vegetable soups		Thickened soups, cream soups
Fish	All white and oily fish (grilled, poached, smoked). Avoid skin (e.g. on sardines or whitebait)	Fish fried in suitable oils	Roe, fish fried in unknown or unsuitable oils or fats
Shellfish	Turkey, chicken, veal, game, rabbit, spring lamb. Very lean beef, ham, bacon, lamb (once or twice a week), Veal or chicken sausage. Liver twice a month	Duck, goose, all visibly fatty meats, usual sausages, salamis, meat pies, pates, poultry skin	

Table 2.2: Food choices for a healthy lipid lowering diet

Meat	Polyunsaturated oils, e.g. sunflower, corn, walnut. Monosaturated oils, (olive-oil, rape-seed oil). Soft (unhydrogenated) margarines rich in monosaturated or polyunsaturated oils, low fat spreads	Roast or chipped potatoes cooked in permitted oils	Roast or chipped potatoes, vegetables or rice fried in unknown or unsuitable oils or fats, potato crisps, oven chips, salted tinned vegetables
Fats	Sorbet, jellies, puddings based on skimmed milk, fruit salad, meringue		Ice cream, puddings, dumplings, sauces based on cream or butter
Fruit and veg-etables		Pastry, biscuits prepared with unsaturated margarine or oils	Commercial pastry, biscuits, commercial pies, snacks and puddings
Desserts	Turkish delight, nougat, boiled sweets	Marzipan, halva	Chocolate, toffees, fudge, coconut bars, butterscotch
Baked foods	Walnuts, almonds, chestnuts	Brazils, cashews, peanuts, pistachios	Coconut, slated nuts
Confec-tionary	Tea, filter or instant coffee, water, calorie free soft drinks	Alcohol, low-fat chocolate drinks	Chocolate drinks, Irish coffee, full fat malted drinks, boiled coffee, ordinary soft drinks
Dressings, flavourings	Pepper, mustard, herbs, spices	Low-fat dressings	Added salt, salad dressings, salad cream, mayonnaise

Source: Wood *et al* (1998)

Wei *et al* (1999) carried out a ten-year longitudinal study involving 25,714 American men, with an average age of 43.8 years. Participants completed questionnaires on demographics, personal and family health history and health habits, which included smoking and physical activity. They also had a physical examination at the start and end of the study. This included measurements of height, weight, blood pressure, lipid and fasting plasma glucose levels. They found that overweight and obese men were more likely to smoke, be sedentary and have higher blood pressure and raised cholesterol and triglyceride levels. Of the obese men, 27% died from cardiovascular disease and 44% died because they were unfit. The authors conclude from their study that physical activity is vital as it reduces the risk of cardiovascular disease, diabetes and hypertension, and lowers cholesterol levels.

Haapanien *et al* (1997) report that there is evidence that a sedentary lifestyle in men is a significant independent risk factor for both CHD and hypertension. Studies have consistently shown the association of physical activity in men and a reduction in the risk of CHD. Haapanien *et al* (1997) report that middle-aged and older men who didn't participate in vigorous activity had a 35% higher incidence of hypertension than those who were more active.

The Exercise Alliance (2001a) provides participation rates of physical activity among people from black and minority ethnic groups. Among African-Caribbean people aged between sixteen and seventy-four years, 32% of men and 31% of women are sedentary compared with 24% of the general population. Among South Asian men in the same age range, 67% of Indians, 72% of Pakistanis and 75% of Bangladeshis do not take part in enough physical activity to benefit their health, compared with 59% of the general population.

Hypertension (high blood pressure)

If you have hypertension, reducing your blood pressure by 5mmHg can reduce your risk of having a heart attack by about 20% (BHF, 2004). Not surprisingly, hypertension is associated with a risk of developing CHD. People with hypertension are three times more likely to develop CHD and stroke and are twice as likely to die from these diseases than those who have normal blood pressure. The higher the blood pressure, the higher the risk (DoH, 2001a). The BHF (2002) report that in England, 41% of men are hypertensive (systolic of 140mmHg or more and a diastolic of 90mmHg or more). The prevalence of hypertension increases with age. Bangladeshi and Chinese men are about 25% less likely to be hypertensive than men in the general population.

The Chief Medical Officer for the DoH reports that 37% of strokes could be prevented if hypertension were treated appropriately (DoH, 2001a). Hypertension can be treated by lifestyle changes such as reducing salt intake; increasing consumption of fruit and vegetables; reducing weight or obesity; and increasing physical activity. In the UK, 75% of our salt intake comes from the consumption of processed foods and so the DoH is working with the food industry to reduce this (DoH, 2001a). The DoH Priorities and Planning Framework for 2002/2003 (2001b) states that one of the NHS Plan's objectives is to reduce deaths from CHD by 40% in people under seventy-five years by 2010 — by meeting the CHD National Standard Framework standards, aiming to improve the health of the worst-off in particular. Building on achievements in 2001, the action for 2002/2003 supports the roll out of action on a health diet particularly targeting deprived areas, including the planned fifty new Five-A-Day community initiatives and the expansion of the school fruit scheme to reach 600,000 children.

Hurst (2002) states that adults should have their blood pressure measured at least every five years. Once hypertension is diagnosed, attention should be paid to exercise, diet, weight and alcohol. In terms of weight, for each kilogram lost, the blood pressure falls by 2.5/1.5 mmHg. A reduction in salt intake of 10g to 5g lowers the blood pressure by 5/3 mmHg. Eating seven portions of fruit and vegetables a day lowers blood pressure in hypertensive patients by 7/3 mmHg and, if combined with a low-fat diet, their blood pressure will fall by 11/6 mmHg.

Sacks *et al* (2001) report on their research study that introduced the Dietary Approaches to Stop Hypertension (DASH) diet. They found that the DASH diet — which advocates fruit, vegetables, low-fat dairy foods and whole grain products, poultry, fish and nuts, and contains reduced amounts of red meat, fats and sugar — lowers blood pressure. Furthermore, combining a reduced salt intake with the DASH diet produced greater reductions in blood pressure.

Smoking

Tobacco use kills around 106,000 people in the UK every year, more than 300 every day — as if a plane crashed every day and killed all of its passengers, around 20% of all deaths.

ASH (2004a)

More men die from smoking each year than were killed during the whole of World War Two. And that's a fact. Low-tar products only con you. All smoking kills — be it from cancer or heart disease. A third of all cancer deaths are linked to smoking.

World Cancer Research Fund (1997: 3)

Box. 2.2: Key facts about smoking

- Smoking has more than fifty ways of making life a misery through illness, and more than twenty ways of killing you.
- About 90% of cases of peripheral vascular disease that lead to amputation of one or both legs are caused by smoking — about 2000 amputations a year in the UK.
- In 2002, 27% of men and 24% of women smoked, which equates to around 12.3 million smokers in the UK. This is a slight decrease on 2001, when 28% of men and 26% of women smoked.
- Smoking kills over 120,000 people in the UK every year.
- Cigarette smoking increases the risk of having a heart attack by two or three times, compared with the risk for non-smokers.
- Smoking causes around one in five deaths from cardiovascular disease.
- Regular exposure to second-hand smoke increases the risk of CHD by about 25%.
- Smoking kills almost six times as many people as road and other accidents; suicide; murder; manslaughter; poisoning; overdoses; and HIV — put together. This is equivalent to a jumbo jet crashing every day of the year, or 3330 people each day, or 120,000 each year.
- Roughly 50% of all smokers will ultimately be killed by their habit.
- Every day in the UK about 450 children start smoking.
- Men under forty-five years of age who smoke twenty-five cigarettes or more a day are fifteen times as likely to die from CHD as non-smokers of the same age.
- People in lower social classes are more likely to die early due to a number of factors. Among men the dominant factor is smoking, which accounts for over 50% of the difference in premature death between social classes.
- Premature deaths from lung cancer are five times higher among men in unskilled manual work than those in professional work.
- In social class I, about 15% of men smoke — compared with about 45% in social class V.
- Households in the lowest tenth of income spend six times as much of their income on tobacco as households in the highest tenth.
- Among those living in the greatest hardship, smoking rates are 70%.
- There is evidence that a smoker's level of nicotine dependence increases systematically with deprivation. Poorer smokers achieve higher intakes of nicotine both by choosing to smoke more cigarettes and by smoking each cigarette more intensively. Since nicotine dependence is an important determinant of ease of quitting, this might be one reason for the lower rates of cessation in those who are more disadvantaged.
- Treating smoking-related illnesses costs the NHS £1.7 billion every year.

⌘ Roughly 75% of regular adult smokers began smoking daily before the age of twenty years (Corrigall *et al*, 2001).

⌘ In Northern Ireland, the 2001 figures showed that 29% of people over the age of sixteen smoked. Men were almost twice as likely (19%) than women (10%) to smoke more than twenty-five cigarettes a day.

Sources: ASH (2004); BHF (2004); DoH (2001a); Corrigall *et al*, 2001

Tobacco smoking is a major determinant of premature mortality and morbidity throughout the world. 'It is estimated that there are currently more than 1.2 billion smokers worldwide, and four million deaths from tobacco annually' (Steptoe *et al*, 2002: 1561). Why is smoking cigarettes so dangerous? According to Cancer Research UK (2002a), 'there are more than 4000 different compounds in tobacco smoke, many of which are toxic; cause cancer; or damage cells.' The three main ingredients are:

1. **Nicotine**: a powerful, fast-acting, addictive drug that causes the 'hit' when drawing on a cigarette. Most of the fifteen million smokers in the UK are addicted to nicotine and crave cigarettes to feed their habit.
2. **Carbon monoxide**: a tasteless, odourless, poisonous gas. It is quickly and easily taken up in the bloodstream once a cigarette is lit.
3. **Tar**: particulate matter composed of a variety of chemicals, many of which are known to cause cancer in animals.

Table 2.3 (*overleaf*) is a list of just some of the 4000 chemicals found in cigarettes and their common uses.

Table 2.3: Some chemicals found in cigarettes and their uses	
Chemical	**Common use**
Acetone	A solvent used in nail-varnish remover
Acetic acid	Vinegar
Ammonia	Used in dry-cleaning agents
Arsenic	A poison found in insecticides
Benzene	Petrol fumes; a known cancer-causing agent used in fuel and chemical manufacture
Cadmium	A highly poisonous metal known to cause liver, kidney and brain damage in humans
Carbon monoxide	Car exhaust fumes
Caesium	A heavy metal
DDT	Insecticide
Ethanol	Antifreeze
Formaldehyde	A highly poisonous liquid found in embalming fluid
Hydrogen cyanide	Industrial pollutant
Hydrogen sulphide	Stink bombs
Lead	Batteries, petrol fumes
Methanol	Rocket fuel
Nicotine	Insecticide
Polonium-210	Radioactive fallout
Radon	Radioactive gas
Sulphuric acid	Power-station emissions
Tars	Road surfaces

Sources: www.roycastle.org/fagends/content.htm (accessed January 2003);
Cancer Research UK (2002a)

Cigarette smoking increases the risk of developing CHD due to its effects on the heart and blood vessels. 'Within one minute of starting to smoke, the heart rate begins to rise: it may increase by as much as 30% during the first ten minutes of smoking. Nicotine raises blood pressure; blood vessels constrict, which forces the heart to work harder to deliver oxygen to the rest of the body. Meanwhile, carbon monoxide in tobacco smoke exerts a negative effect on the heart by reducing the blood's ability to carry oxygen' (ASH, 2002: 1).

It is estimated that about 20% of male deaths from CHD are due to cigarette smoking. It is suggested that the prevalence of males who smoke cigarettes in the UK in 1998 was 28%. Furthermore, it was estimated that 9% of boys aged eleven to fifteen years were regular smokers, with 'regular' being defined as smoking a minimum of one cigarette per week. Since the 1970s, it has been noted that the prevalence of adults smoking and the number of cigarettes smoked has been falling — but the decline now seems to be levelling off. In Britain today, it is suggested that 40% of men aged twenty-five to thirty-four smoke regularly (Cancer Research UK, 2002a). Men under forty-five years of age who smoke twenty-five cigarettes or more per day are fifteen times more likely to die from CHD than their non-smoking counterparts (ASH, 2002). Once again, there seem to be geographical differences, with both adults and teenagers in Scotland and Northern Ireland smoking more than those in England and Wales. In England, smoking rates tend to be higher in the north than in the south.

Smoking is the principal cause of the inequalities in death rates between the rich and poor. Put simply, smoking is a public-health disaster.

Alan Milburn, UK Secretary of State for Health (1999–2003)

Manual workers tend to smoke more than non-manual workers. The BHF (2002) reports that 36% of men in manual occupations smoke, compared with 21% in non-manual occupations. The UK Government's Cancer Plan aims to reduce smoking in the 'manual classes' to 26% by 2010 (Cancer Research, 2002a). Bancroft *et al* (2003: 1261) note that the relationship between smoking and socioeconomic factors is particularly marked: 'The 1998 Scottish Health Survey indicated that 45% of men and 56% of women in Social Class V smoked, compared with 12% and 11%, respectively, in Social Class I.' Bancroft *et al* (2003) also note that in order to maximise the effect of nicotine, poorer people smoke more cigarettes, and do so more intensely.

There is also an ethnic variation in smoking rates, particularly raised in Bangladeshi men (42%); Irish men (39%) and Caribbean men (42%). Smith *et al* (2000: 399) suggest that religion may have an influence on rates of smoking in ethnic groups since, 'religious limits are placed on smoking among Sikhs ... absence of a Muslim prohibition on smoking, although there is a general expectation of restraint for women'.

Box. 2.3: Key facts about smoking in young men

⌘ One in ten teenagers in the UK regularly smokes cigarettes. By age fifteen years, more than one in five smokes regularly.

⌘ It is estimated that in 2004 there were around 375,000 regular smokers aged eleven-to-fifteen in the UK.

⌘ Young people are seven times less likely to smoke if their parents disapprove strongly of smoking, even if they smoke themselves.

⌘ Three out of four children are aware of cigarettes before they reach the age of five years, whether their parents smoke or not.

⌘ It is very rare for someone to take up smoking as an adult; the majority of smokers start during adolescence. Ninety-five percent of smokers started as children.

⌘ In the early 1980s, boys and girls were equally likely to smoke. Since then, girls have been consistently more likely to smoke than boys.

⌘ Smoking has been shown to have a strong relationship with social and educational characteristics. Prevalence of smoking is higher among those who are socially disadvantaged.

⌘ Schoolchildren who smoke are also likely to drink alcohol and/or take drugs.

Sources: www.roycastle.org/kats/facts_stats.htm;
Boreham and Shaw (2001); Peterson and Peto (2004)

All teenagers who smoke tend to have certain general characteristics:

- they have family members and friends who smoke
- they are more likely to come from single-parent families
- they may have low self-esteem, low confidence, more anxiety and poor educational aspirations
- their leisure time is spent working part-time or 'hanging about'

Source: Coleman and Hendry (1999)

By 2030, tobacco is expected to be the single biggest preventable cause of premature death and disease worldwide.

(Sandford 2003: 7)

Switching to lower tar cigarettes is also of little benefit, as the evidence suggests that smokers of low-tar cigarettes simply inhale more deeply or cover up the filter holes with their fingers to get the same hit. As a result, some highly dangerous forms of lung cancer actually appear to be higher in smokers of low-tar cigarettes.

www.malehealth.co.uk/userpage1.cfm?item_id=154
(accessed January 2005)

Someone who has never smoked is 60% less likely than someone who has smoked to develop CHD and is 30% less likely to have a stroke. Deciding not to smoke is equivalent to choosing life against chronic ill-health and premature death.

(DoH, 1999)

There is no simple way to prevent young people starting to smoke. School-based programmes have limited success, although social reinforcement/social norms-type programmes seem to be more effective than traditional knowledge-based interventions.

(NCRD, 1999)

Aveyard *et al* (2003) carried out a cluster randomised controlled trial to examine whether disengagement from an adolescent smoking prevention and cessation intervention was an independent risk factor for regular smoking one and two years later. Their sample consisted of 8352 thirteen to fourteen year-old school pupils from the West Midlands, UK. In the study, the intervention group was asked to use an interactive computer programme on three separate occasions. (It is known that health promotion interventions are not successful unless people engage with them.) Aveyard *et al* (2003) found that pupils who disengaged from the school-based health promotion programme were more likely to smoke cigarettes.

The benefits of not starting to smoke in the first place are clear. Someone who has never smoked is 60% less likely than someone who has smoked to develop CHD, and is 30% less likely to have a stroke. Deciding not to smoke is equivalent to choosing life against chronic ill-health and premature death (DoH, 1999). By 2030, tobacco is expected to be the single biggest preventable cause of premature death and disease worldwide (Sandford, 2003).

Advantages of giving up smoking

Stopping smoking cuts the risk of a heart attack to about half that of a smoker within one year, and after a number of years the risk is the same as someone who has never smoked.

(Peterson and Peto, 2002: 4)

> *Stopping smoking soon after a heart attack reduces the risk of dying of a subsequent attack by 25%.*
>
> (Peterson and Peto, 2004: 6)

Giving up smoking, particularly before the age of thirty, immediately cuts down the risks of developing lung cancer, CHD, bronchitis and emphysema. Stopping smoking will almost certainly increase the length of your life. You will also:

- ⌘ Feel fitter and perform better — including in the bedroom. Smoking reduces the quality and, owing to reduced blood flow, the size of male erections. It also damages sperm.
- ⌘ Look and smell better.
- ⌘ Be able to taste good food and smell sweet smells again.
- ⌘ Be richer — in the UK, a twenty-a-day cigarette habit costs well over £1,000 a year.
- ⌘ Be doing everyone a favour — if you have children, you will no longer be a health hazard to them or to the rest of the population.

> Source: http://www.malehealth.co.uk/userpage1.cfm?item_id=154# advantages (accessed January 2005)

Tips for quitting smoking

1. Make a date to stop smoking and stick to it. Most people who quit smoking do it by quitting altogether and not by gradually cutting down.
2. Think positively about the withdrawal symptoms you experience when you stop smoking. These are very good signs because they signal that your body is recovering from the effects of tobacco. They will disappear in a week or two.
3. Change your routine so as to avoid situations in which you will get a strong urge to smoke. The more you change your routine, the easier it will be to stop.
4. Drink lots of water.
5. Become more active as this will help you to relax.
6. Start saving money by putting away the amount you would have spent on tobacco or cigarettes per week or month.
7. Treat yourself by using the money you have saved by stopping smoking.
8. Watch what you eat if you are worried about putting on weight. Rather than snacking, eat some fruit or chew some sugar-free gum.
9. Take one day at a time.

10. Make no excuses — don't use a crisis or a special occasion as an excuse for 'just one' cigarette.

Source: http://www.cancer.ie/quitting/tips.php (accessed January 2005)

What to do if you get a craving or urge to have a cigarette

⌘ Take deep breaths — slowly inhale and exhale.
⌘ Drink some water.
⌘ Do something else — shopping, go for a walk, call a friend.
⌘ Dip into your alternatives — whether it's a carrot, nicotine gum, or a boiled sweet.
⌘ Most of all, delay reaching for a cigarette — the body will readjust, so the worst craving only lasts a short while.

Source: http://www.malehealth.co.uk/userpage1.cfm?item_id=154# advantages (accessed January 2005)

There are a variety of UK government and EU initiatives being introduced to stress the 'stop smoking' message. Sandford (2003) lists these as being the requirement to increase the size of health warnings on cigarette packets by 30% and banning the use of misleading terms such as 'light' and 'mild'. 'Norway and Finland were among the first countries to ban advertising and there was a noticeable decline in smoking rates after the implementation of legislation' (Sandford, 2003: 10).

In the UK, the annual 'No Smoking Day', now in its twentieth year, is seen as particularly successful: typical figures are that about one million smokers attempt to quit as a result, with some 400,000 managing to quit in the longer term. The use of telephone helplines in smoking cessation is helpful, but as Sandford (2003) points out (*Table 2.4*), the combined effect of available aids is the most effective method.

'Stopping smoking never killed anybody, but continuing to smoke kills 300 people every day in the UK' (Steet, 2002: 1). Steet (2002) provides some interesting information regarding the benefits of smoking cessation:

- nicotine disappears within eight hours
- carbon monoxide disappears within twenty-four hours
- over time, 4200 chemicals present in tobacco smoke disappear
- after twelve months of stopping smoking, insurance companies class individuals as non-smokers
- not smoking twenty cigarettes a day saves £1000 per year.

Table 2.4: Smoking interventions and their effectiveness	
Intervention used	**Proportion of smokers making an attempt to stop who will be abstinent after 12 months**
Tries to stop using will power alone	3%
Tries to stop using self-help materials (ie. audiotapes, videos, booklets)	4%
Tries to stop using NRT bought from a pharmacy	6%
Tries to stop with the help of a smokers' clinic, but without NRT	10%
Tries to stop with the help of a smokers' clinic and NRT bought from a pharmacy	20%

Passive smoking is also a risk factor for CHD. Josefson (2001) reports that even transient, short-term exposure to environmental smoke significantly reduces coronary blood flow in healthy young non-smokers. The American Lung Association estimates that between 35,000 and 50,000 deaths per year are attributable to passive smoking. Peterson and Peto (2004) state that a non-smoker who lives with a smoker increases their risk of developing CHD by 23%. In the UK, it is estimated that there may be as many as 12,000 cases of heart disease every year which can be attributed to passive smoking. According to ASH (2002: 1), 'there is now evidence that passive smoking is associated with increased risk of stroke in men and women.' Norway, Ireland and Italy have all banned smoking in public places (bars restaurants, cafes, pubs and clubs) to reduce the risks of passive (or second hand smoke) on both employees and consumers. Scotland plans to follow in 2006.

Weight and obesity

> *Carry an extra 50lbs of body fat and you're 700% more likely to develop hypertension, 3000% more likely to develop diabetes, more likely to develop prostate cancer, colon cancer and rectal cancer. Obesity will kill you! Even moderate overweight is a big cause of almost all disease and health problems. It damages the immune system, reducing your resistance to everything.*
>
> http://www.man-health-magazine-online.com/health-man.html

Being overweight or obese increases the risk of CHD and developing type 2 diabetes (Adolfsson *et al*, 2005). The risk is greater if the excess weight is concentrated in the abdominal area. The latter is termed 'central obesity'. The rate of obesity in men (22%) in the UK has tripled since the mid-1980s. The trend is also increasing in children, with 22% of boys and 28% of girls being overweight or obese. In countries where statistics are available, the UK now has one of the fastest growing rates of obesity; only Kuwait and Samoa are above the UK rate (BHF, 2004).

Body mass index (BMI)

Your BMI is an indicator of your weight. BMI can be calculated by dividing body weight (kg) by the square of height (m^2). The ideal range of BMI for adults is 20–25 kg/m^2. A person is overweight if their BMI is over 25 and obese if it's over 30 (BNF, 2001). The likelihood of being overweight and obese increases with age. In the age group 16–24 years, 28% of men are overweight or obese compared with 76% in the age group 55–64 years. Central obesity also increases with age, particularly in men. In men over 55 years of age, the rate is about 46% compared with 7% in the 16–34 age range. In men, a waist circumference greater or equal to 94 cm is an indication of the need to lose weight, and a measurement greater or equal to 102 cm requires the individual to receive professional advice on weight reduction (Wood *et al*, 1998). The rates of being overweight and obese have been increasing in the last couple of decades. The percentage of adults who are obese is about double the rate in the 1980s and the high levels of being overweight and obese in children are likely to increase further. Both sexes in unskilled occupations are over four times as likely as those in professional employment to be classed as morbidly obese (BMI>40) (BHF, 2002).

Levels of obesity are lower in Pakistani, Indian, Chinese and, most markedly, Bangladeshi men, who are three times less likely to be obese than men in the general population. Despite lower levels of general obesity, central obesity levels are higher in Pakistani, Bangladeshi and Indian men, with the latter group having a rate of 41% compared with 28% of men in the general population.

Diabetes mellitus

Diabetes substantially increases the risk of CHD. It is estimated that there are about 1.3 million people with diagnosed diabetes in the UK and that nearly 50% of diabetes cases may be undiagnosed. Men with non-insulin dependent diabetes have between two and four times the risk of CHD than those who are not diabetic. The incidence of diabetes increases with age. The prevalence of diagnosed diabetes has increased by 65% in men since 1991. The rate of non-insulin treated diabetes in men in low socioeconomic groups is about 36% higher than in more affluent groups. The prevalence of diabetes in Pakistani and Bangladeshi men is fives times greater than in the general population, and two-and-a-half times greater in Black Caribbean men than in the general population (BHF, 2004).

Psychosocial well-being

There is a link between psychosocial well-being and the development of coronary heart disease. Four areas are highlighted as being particularly involved: depression, social support, work-related stress and personality type. Working in jobs with a high level of stress and/or a lack of control increases the risk of developing CHD and dying prematurely. Poor social support can have a detrimental effect on health and recovering from illness (DoH, 1999).

One way of measuring levels of depression, anxiety, sleep disturbance and happiness is to use the General Health Questionnaire (GHQ12), which has proven to be a valid and reliable tool. Gaining a score of four of more indicates a high level of psychological distress. Women tend to have a slightly higher score than men (18% compared with 13%) and the scores tend to be higher in both sexes aged over seventy-five years. Individuals with a low income tend to have a higher score indicating psychological distress than those with higher incomes. The BHF (2002) report that Bangladeshis have the highest levels of psychological distress, followed by Pakistanis. Some 28% of Bangladeshi men have high levels of psychological distress.

Men are more likely to report a lack of social support, which is strongly linked with social class. Both sexes in social class V are twice as likely to report a severe lack of social support compared with those in social class 1. South Asian, Chinese and Black Caribbean people are more likely to report a severe lack of social support. In men, 41% of Chinese and 37% of Bangladeshis fall into this category (BHF, 2004).

Alcohol

Alcohol is believed to be associated with reduced risk of CHD, but only if taken in moderation (one or two drinks per day). If those levels are exceeded or people indulge in binge drinking, then the risk is greater. BHF (2002) state that 38% of men consume more alcohol than the recommended levels of between three and four units per day. Men are twice as likely to be heavy drinkers than women. Proctor (2003) states that the latest figures from the Office of National Statistics show that 27% of men and 15% of women drink more than the recommended limits. He also cites Alcohol Concern's suggestion that one in thirteen of Britain's adult population is alcohol-dependent.

There is evidence too of age differences: in younger age groups, 50% of men in the sixteen-to-twenty-four years age group drink more than the recommended levels compared with 16% of men over sixty-five years of age. Again, there are regional and sex differences, with the highest rate of excessive alcohol intake in men in Merseyside and the north-east of England, and the lowest in London and the South East. Irish men and women are more likely to exceed recommended levels than those in the general population with 74% of Irish men reported to exceed the guidelines on the heaviest drinking day. Smith *et al* (2000: 399) suggest that religion may have an influence on drinking alcohol in ethnic groups, since 'religious limits are placed on... drinking alcohol among Muslims... Sikh male levels of drinking reflect the absence of specific Sikh prohibition on alcohol'.

Health promotion and preventative care

According to Cappuccio *et al* (2002), the prevention of CHD relies on a reduction of overall absolute risk of the disease rather than the management of individual risk factors. Therefore, preventative measures should be directed towards lifestyle changes and, where appropriate, drug therapies (Wood *et al*, 1998). Song and Lee (2001: 376) argue that individuals have to be motivated to take advantage of health-related knowledge and facilities. They define motivation as 'a process that is directed toward a future goal and an integrative process of goal setting and self-evaluative reaction.'

To prevent CHD, a healthy diet is one that is low in salt and transfatty acids, and low in dietary cholesterol. The Mediterranean diet is an example of this. The traditional Japanese diet is low in fat and high in complex carbohydrates. Both these diets are associated with the best life expectancy in the world (Wood *et al*, 1998).

Screening plays a part in preventing CHD in the families of those who already have the disease. Wood *et al* (1998) recommend that close relatives of those who have premature CHD (under fifty-five years of age in men) should be screened for CHD, as they too are at risk of developing the disease.

The DoH (1999) set out actions for reducing the risk of CHD or stroke, outlined below:

- Major changes in diet, particularly among the worst off, with increased consumption of such foods as fruit, vegetables and oily fish.
- Large reductions in tobacco smoking, particularly among young people, women, and people in disadvantaged communities.
- People keeping more physically active — by walking briskly or cycling, for example — on a regular basis.
- People controlling their body weight so as to keep to the right level for their physique.

⌘   Avoiding drinking alcohol to excess.

The UK government, in its white paper *Smoking Kills* (1998), set out policies for addressing smoking as one of the major causes of stroke and CHD. They set up a three-year public education campaign costing up to £50 million; banned tobacco advertising; and set aside £60 million, to be spent over three years, for smoking cessation services in deprived areas known as Health Action Zones.

The BNF (2004) recommends the following:

⌘   Maintain a healthy body weight (BMI 20–25kg/m^2).
⌘   Keep physically active.
⌘   Eat less fat and fewer fatty foods.
⌘   Use vegetable oil that is high in unsaturated fat in cooking, but only in small amounts — eg. olive oil or rapeseed oil.
⌘   Eat more fruits and vegetables — at least five portions a day.
⌘   Eat more starchy foods like potatoes, rice, pasta, bread and breakfast cereals.
⌘   Choose high-fibre wholemeal products.
⌘   Eat fish at least twice a week, of which one portion should be oily fish.
⌘   Choose lean meat, poultry, beans and alternatives instead of fatty meat or meat products.
⌘   Choose low-fat dairy foods, like skimmed or semi-skimmed milk, or low-fat yoghurt.
⌘   Choose low-salt products and use less salt in cooking.
⌘   Drink moderately — the recommendations are three to four units per day for men and two to three units per day for women.

Making changes to one's lifestyle, such as those recommended above, is a complex issue involving lay understandings of disease and its causes, risk and a range of socioeconomic factors (Wiles and Kinmonth, 2001).

Useful websites (all last accessed January 2005)

Angina — www.angina.org.uk
Asian Tobacco Education Campaign — www.ash.orh.uk/html/cessation/
    asianeducation.pdf
Blood Pressure Association — www.bpassoc.org.uk
British Heart Foundation — www.bhf.org.uk
National Heart Forum — www.heartforum.org.uk
Quit — stopsmoking@quit.org.uk; online counselling service for people trying to stop
    smoking
WHO Europe — www.who.dk

References

Adolfsson B, Andersson I, Elofsson S, Rossner S, Unden AL (2005) Locus of control
    and weight reduction. *Patient Educ Counsel* **56**: 55–61
Alcohol Concern (2001) The State of the Nation: Britain's True Alcohol Bill.
www.alcoholconcern.org.uk (last accessed January 2005)
ASH (2004) Smoking and Disease. www.ash.org.uk/html/factsheets/html/basic02.html
    (accessed January 2005)
Aveyard P, Marham WA, Almond J, Lancashire E, Cheng KK (2003) The risk of
    smoking in relation to engagement with a school-based smoking intervention.
    Soc Sci Med **56**: 869–82
Bancroft A, Wiltshire S, Parry O, Amos A (2003) 'It's like an addiction first thing…
    afterwards it's like a habit': daily smoking behaviour among people living in
    areas of deprivation. *Soc Sci Med* **56**: 1261–7
Boreham R, Shaw A (eds) (2001) *Smoking, Drinking and Drug Use Among Young
    People in England in 2000*. Norwich: HMSO
British Heart Foundation (2004) BHF 2004 Coronary Heart Disease Statistics.
    http://www.bhf.org.uk/news/uploaded/fact_sheet2.pdf (accessed January 2005)
British Nutrition Foundation (BNF) (2004) Heart Disease and Stroke (Cardiovacular
    Disease). http://www.nutrition.org.uk/home.asp?siteId=43&sectionId=404&subSe
    ctionId=321&parentSection=299&which=1 (accessed January 2005)
Cancer Research UK (2002a) Smoking and Cancer. www.cancerresearchuk.org
    September 2002
Cappuccio FP, Oakeshott P, Strazzullo P, Kerry SM (2002) Application of Framington
    risk estimates to ethnic minorities in United Kingdom and implications
    for primary prevention of heart disease in general practice: cross-sectional
    population-based study. *BMJ* **325**: 1271–6
Chief Medical Officer (2001) *The Health of the Public in Northern Ireland*. Belfast.

Coleman JC, Hendry LB (1999) *Adolescent Health.* 3rd ed. London: Routledge

Corrigall WA, Zack M, Eissenberg T, Belsito L, Scher R (2001) Acute subjective and physiological responses to smoking in adolescents. *Addiction* **96**: 1409–17

Department of Health (DoH) (1994) *Nutritional Aspects of Cardiovascular Disease. Report of the Cardiovascular Review Group of the Committee on Medical Aspects of Food Policy (COMA).* London: HMSO

DoH (1998) *Smoking Kills – A White Paper on Tobacco.* Executive summary at http://www.doh.gov.uk/smokexec.htm (last accessed January 2005)

DoH (1999) *Saving Lives: Our Healthier Nation.* London: HMSO

DoH (2000) National Service Framework for Coronary Heart Disease. http://www.dh.gov.uk/PolicyAndGuidance/HealthAndSocialCareTopics/ CoronaryHeartDisease/fs/en (last accessed January 2005)

DoH (2001a) *The Annual Report of the Chief Medical Officer of the Department of Health 2001: On the State of the Public Health.* London: HMSO

DoH (2001b) Priorities and Planning Framework 2002/2003. http://www.doh.gov.uk/ planning2002-2003/index.htm (last accessed January 2005)

Exercise Alliance (2001) www.exercisealliance.org.uk (accessed April 2002)

The Financial Times (2003) Norway bans public smoking. 10 April: 7. www.health-news.co.uk (accessed April 2003)

Haapanen N, Miilunpalo S, Vuori I, Oja P, Pasanen M (1997) Association of leisure time physical activity with the risk of coronary heart disease, hypertension and diabetes in middle-aged men and women. *Int J Epidemiol* **26**(4): 739–47

Hemingway H, Marmot M (1999) Psychological factors in the aetiology and prognosis of coronary heart disease: a systematic review of prospective cohort studies. *BMJ* **318**: 1460–7

Hunt K, Davison C, Emslie C, Ford G (2000) Are perceptions of a family history of heart disease related to health-related attitudes and behaviour? *Health Educ Res* **15**(2): 131–43

Hurst R (2002) Managing hypertension: measurement and prevention. *Nurs Times* **98**(38): 38–40

Inchley J, Todd J, Bryce C, Currie C (2001) Dietary trends among Scottish schoolchildren in the 1990s. *J Hum Nutr Diet* **14**: 207–16

Josefson D (2001) Study links passive smoking and coronary blood flow. *BMJ* 323: 252

Kivimaki M, Leino-Arjas P, Luukkonen R, Riihimaki H, Vahtera J, Kirjonen J (2002) Work stress and risk of cardiovascular mortality: prospective cohort study of industrial employees. *BMJ* **325**: 857–61

Lloyd T, Forrest S (2001) *Boy's and Young Men's Health: Literature and Practice Review.* London: Health Development Agency

Macintyre K, Stewart S, Chalmers J, Pell J, Finlayson A, Boyd J, Redpath A, McMurray J, Capewell S (2001) Relation between socioeconomic deprivation and death from a first myocardial infarction in Scotland: population-based analysis. *BMJ* **322**: 1152–1523

NHS Centre for Reviews and Dissemination (NCRD) (1999) Preventing the uptake of smoking in young people. *Eff Health Care* **5**(5): 1–12

Office for National Statistics (2000) *Living in Great Britain: Results from the 1998 General Household Survey.* London: HMSO

Peterson S, Peto V (2004) Smoking Statistics. British Heart Foundation Health Promotion Research Group, Department of Public Health. http://www.heartstats. org/datapage.asp?id=3916 (accessed January 2005)

Primatesta P (1998) Prevalence of cardiovascular disease. http://www.archive. official-documents.co.uk/document/doh/survey98/hse-02.htm (last accessed January 2005)

Proctor D (2003) Alcohol-related health problems in general hospitals. *Nurs Times* **99**(9): 26–7

Richardson DP (2000) The grain, the wholegrain and nothing but the grain: the science behind wholegrain and the reduced risk of heart disease and cancer. *British Nutrition Foundation Nutrition Bulletin* **25**: 353–60

Sacks FM, Svetkey LP, Vollmer WM, Appel LJ, Bray GA, Hasha D, Obarzanek E, Conlin PR, Miller ER, Simons-Morton DG, Karanja N, Lin PH (2001) Effects on blood pressure of reduced dietary sodium and the dietary approaches to stop hypertension (DASH) diet. *New Engl J Med* **344**: 3–10

Sandford A (2003) Government action to reduce smoking. *Respirology* **8**: 7–16

Scottish Office Department of Health (1998) *Working Together for a Healthier Scotland.* Edinburgh: SODH

Smith GD, Chaturvedi N, Harding S, Nazroo J, Williams R (2000) Ethnic inequalities in health: a review of UK epidemiological evidence. *Critical Public Health* **10**(4): 375–408

Song R, Lee H (2001) Managing health habits for myocardial infarction (MI) patients. *Int J Nurs Stud* **38**: 375–80

Steet C (2002) Stop smoking. Medicom. http://www.glosgoodhealth.org.uk/smoking. htm (accessed January 2005)

Steptoe A, Wardle J, Cui W, Baban A, Glass K, Pelzer K, Tsuda A, Vinck J (2002) An international comparison of tobacco smoking, beliefs and risk awareness in university students from 23 countries. *Addiction* **97**: 1561–71

Tod AM, Read C, Lacey A, Abbott J (2001) Barriers to uptake of services for coronary heart disease: qualitative study. *BMJ* **323**: 1–6

Wallis EJ, Ramsey LE, Haq IU, Ghahramani P, Jackson PR, Rowland-Yeo K, Yeo WW (2000) Coronary and cardiovascular risk estimation for primary prevention: validation of a new Sheffield table in the 1995 Scottish health survey population. *BMJ* **320**: 671–6

Wanless D (2002) *Securing Our Future Health: Taking a Long-term View. Final Report.* London: HM Treasury

Wei M, Kamper JB, Barlow CE, Nichaman MZ, Gibbons LW, Paffenbarger RS, Blair SN (1999) Relationship between low cardiorespiratory fitness and mortality in normal-weight, overweight and obese men. *JAMA* **282**: 1547–53

WHO (2001) Cardiovascular Diseases: Prevention and Control. World Health Organisation. www.who.int/ncd/cvd/index.htm (accessed January 2005)

Wiles R, Kinmonth A (2001) Patients' understandings of heart attack: implications for prevention of recurrence. *Patient Education and Counselling* **44**: 161–9

Wood D, de Backer G, Faergeman O, Graham I, Mancia G, Pyorala K (1998) Prevention of coronary heart disease in clinical practice: recommendations of the Second Joint Task Force of European and Other Societies on Coronary Prevention. *Eur Heart J* **19**: 1434–1503

Woolf-May K, Kearney EM, Owen A, Jones DW, Davison RCR, Bird SR (1999) The efficacy of accumulates short bouts versus single daily bouts of brisk walking in improving aerobic fitness and blood lipid profiles. *Health Educ Res* **14**(6): 803–15

World Cancer Research Fund (1997) *One Careful Owner. Preventing Cancer: What Every Man Should Know*. London: WCRF

Chapter 3

Cancers and other diseases predominantly affecting men

One in three people will get cancer at some time in their lives, and one in four will die from the disease. There are over 260,000 new cases each year, of which just over half affect men.

www.malehealth.co.uk/userpage1.cfm?item_id=117 (accessed January 2005)

Deaths from cancer account for 26% of all male deaths.

Wanless (2002: 22)

Cancer has now overtaken coronary heart disease as the commonest cause of death in Scotland.

Scottish Executive (2001: 16)

There were an estimated 2.6 million new cases of cancer in Europe in 1995, representing over one-quarter of the world burden of cancer. The corresponding number of deaths from cancer was approximately 1.6 million... In men, the most common primary sites were lung (22% of all cancer cases), colon and rectum (12%), and prostate (11%).

Bray *et al* (2001: 99)

According to www.malehealth.co.uk, using the UK government's Office of National Statistics, the odds for men for the three most common cancers are:

12–1: lung cancer (55–1 before the age of sixty-five years)
13–1: prostate cancer (111–1 before age sixty-five)
18–1: colorectal cancer (71–1 before age sixty-five)

From available statistics, it is reported that Irish men have excess mortality rates for all cancers compared with men in the rest of the UK: 'The mortality from lung cancer in the Irish-born was either highest for all people in England and Wales or second to Scottish people' (Lees and Papadopoulos, 2000: 223).

Box 3.1: Key facts about cancer in men

⌘ Each year in the UK, there are over 127,000 cases of cancer diagnosed in men.

⌘ There are more than 200 different types of cancer, but four of them — lung, breast, colorectal and prostate — account for over half of new cases.

⌘ During their lifetimes, one in three men will be diagnosed with cancer.

⌘ The most commonly diagnosed cancer in men is lung, followed by prostate and bowel cancer.

⌘ In the UK, around 27,000 men are diagnosed with prostate cancer each year. More than 80% of diagnoses are in men aged over seventy years.

⌘ The lifetime risk of prostate cancer is one in fourteen.

⌘ Testicular cancer is the most common cancer in men between the ages of twenty and thirty-five.

⌘ The lifetime risk for being diagnosed with testicular cancer is one in 500.

⌘ There has been a 63% rise in the incidence of prostate cancer, much of which is due to increased detection.

⌘ There has been an 84% rise in the incidence of testicular cancer, but the cause is unknown.

⌘ The male lifetime risk for dying from cancer is one in four.

⌘ Lung cancer is the biggest cause of death from cancer in men in the UK. This is followed by prostate and bowel cancer which, together, account for half of all male deaths from cancer.

Sources: Cancer Research UK (2002b); Carlisle (2002);
Institute of Cancer Research (2005)

Development of cancer

Cancer is a broad term. It is used to describe over 200 diseases, which can affect any part of the body:

Simply speaking, it is a disease of cells, and every type of cancer starts in the same way. It begins when the genetic information in a single cell becomes damaged in some way and causes the cell to divide at an uncontrolled rate. The resulting group of cells forms a lump or swelling — which is usually referred to as a 'tumour'. The tumour may then grow and go on to damage surrounding healthy

*tissues or organs, or cancer cells may break away from the original
tumour and spread through the bloodstream or the lymphatic system
to other parts of the body — a process known as metastasis.*

World Cancer Research Fund www.wcrf.org.uk (accessed December 2002)

*The development of cancer is a complex and curious biological
process, so one single factor is unlikely to be the cause. Hormones,
immune conditions and inherited mutations (alterations) in the genes
of a cell can all have a role in cancer development, but the main
causes are environmental in nature. Environmental factors include
exposure to: toxins, such as tobacco and alcohol; the food we eat;
infectious agents, such as certain viruses and bacteria; chemical
agents, such as asbestos and benzene; and radiation from sunlight
and radioactive materials.'All of these can be 'carcinogenic' — that
is, they can damage and/or alter the normal programming of cells
in the body and so encourage the development of cancer. According
to Hecht (2002), a carcinogen is 'any agent — chemical, physical
or viral — that causes cancer or increases the incidence of cancer'.
Among the 4000 identified chemicals in cigarette smoke, more than
sixty are established carcinogens... These chemical carcinogens are
the cause of cancer from cigarette smoke.*

(Hecht, 2002: 462)

*We also know that cell damage is a cumulative process, and that
'free-radicals', the by-products of normal bodily processes, play a
part in causing this damage. It's thought that certain factors may act
together or in a sequence to initiate and promote the cancer process.
Cancer can take ten to twenty years to develop, which is why it
predominantly affects older people. But it is also why we can take
positive steps to prevent or halt the various stages involved. That's
why diet and lifestyle are so important'*

(World Cancer Research Fund, 1999: 4)

Most cancers are probably caused by a combination of a genetic susceptibility
and a cancer-causing trigger (*Box 3.2*).

Box 3.2: Major causes of cancer

⌘ Smoking — the biggest single cause by far. It's implicated in a third of all cancer deaths and nine out of ten cases of lung cancer.

⌘ Drinking alcohol — some cancers, such as those of the mouth, throat and liver, are linked to excessive alcohol consumption.

⌘ Poor diet — about a quarter of cancers in the UK are related to what we eat. Eating too much fat (particularly animal fat), too little fibre and not enough vitamins can increase the risk of cancer. Vitamins A, C and E are particularly important — these are antioxidants, substances that help neutralise cell-damaging molecules known as free radicals.

⌘ Being overweight — one American study found that people who are obese have a 33% greater risk of cancer.

⌘ The sun — a natural source of radiation and the major cause of the most common cancer, skin cancer.

⌘ Chemicals — pesticides and fungicides are in the dock over some cancers; radon gas and phthalates (found in plastic food containers and clingfilm, as well as vinyl floor tiles and carpet tiles) over others. Pollutants such as benzene and invisible particulates in the air are also carcinogenic, although the exact link between pollution and cancer is unclear.

⌘ Family history — about one in three cancer patients have a close relative who has the disease. Cancers that appear to run most often in families include bowel (25% of cases are hereditary), testicular, prostate, skin and breast cancers.

⌘ Age — the risk of cancer increases as you get older. As a rule of thumb, risk doubles for every decade over the age of twenty-five.

Source: http://www.malehealth.co.uk/userpage1.cfm?item_id=117# whatcausesit
(accessed January 2005)

Tobacco

> *A thought can lead to an action*
> *An action can form a habit*
> *A habit forms a character*
> *A character forms a destiny*
>
> www.roycastle.org (accessed January 2003)

According to Levi (1999), between 25% and 30% of all cancer deaths in Europe are due to tobacco smoking and between 80% and 90% of lung cancers in men are attributable to cigarette smoking. In Europe, roughly one in three adult males are current smokers.

In the UK, only 10% of women and 12% of men in the highest socioeconomic group are smokers, whereas in the lowest socioeconomic group, the corresponding figures are more than three times as high. In every country in Europe, unemployed people are more likely to smoke than those who are employed (WHO, 2001). The most deprived areas in Scotland are associated with the highest risk of being diagnosed with cancer and the lowest chance of survival. At present, among Scots aged between sixteen and seventy-four, 34% of males and 32% of females are regular smokers (Scottish Executive, 2001). 'At a more local level, in a street with 150 adults, of which about forty-five smoke, about twenty will be killed by their smoking' (NHS Health Scotland and ASH Scotland, 2004).

Alcohol

Although alcohol is not a known carcinogen, the risk of cancers of the upper digestive and respiratory tract is increased when individuals drink alcohol and smoke. 'The relative risk of these neoplasms is increased several dozen times in heavy smokers and heavy drinkers' (Levi, 1999: 1918).

Occupational and environmental factors

Estimates of the proportion of cancer deaths attributable to occupational and environmental carcinogens are complex and difficult for any specific population, apart perhaps from the effect of past occupational exposure to asbestos, which may account by itself for 50% of all occupational cancer deaths. Projections for the period 1995–2029 suggest that the number of men dying from mesothelioma in Western Europe each year will almost double over the next twenty years from more than 5000 in 1989 to at least 10,000 around 2018 and then decline, with a total of approximately 250,000 deaths over the next thirty-five years. The highest risk will be suffered by men born around 1945–1950, of whom approximately one in 150 will die of mesothelioma. Asbestos use in Western Europe remained high until about 1980 and substantial quantities are still used in several European countries.

Levi (1999: 1921)

Asbestos and tobacco smoke act together to increase the risk of developing lung cancer (www.cancerbacup.org.uk/info/lung/lung-4.htm accessed January 2005). According to Medicine.Net, asbestos insulation workers have ninety-two times the risk of developing lung cancer compared with the general population, and smelter workers have three-to-eight times the risk (www.focusoncancer. com/script/main/art.asp?li=MNI&ArticleKey=406 accessed January 2005).

General warning signs of cancer

General warning signs are listed by the World Cancer Research Fund UK (www.wcrf-uk.org/publications/ last accessed February 2005) as:

- a noticeable change in bowel or bladder habits for no apparent reason
- a sore or bruise that does not heal as normal
- unusual bleeding or discharge
- a thickening or lump in the breast, testicle or anywhere else in the body
- persistent indigestion or difficulty swallowing
- a significant change, in size or colour, of a wart or mole
- a persistent nagging cough or hoarseness

Preventing cancer

'The old saying: "an ounce of prevention is worth a pound of cure" perfectly describes the benefits of cancer prevention through diet and lifestyle. Not every case of cancer can be controlled in this way, but healthier diets can have a drastic impact on cancer incidence and mortality rates in this country and throughout the world' (World Cancer Research Fund, 2002; www.wcrf-uk.org).

According to Cancer Research UK, 'recently, researchers have suggested that we may be able to prevent as many as thirty-five out of every 100 cases of cancer by altering our diets. However, it is difficult to be exact. Other researchers have suggested a range of figures from 10% to 70% of cancers are preventable by changing diet (www.cancerhelp.org.uk accessed December 2004).

Lees and Papadopoulos (2000) report that the 'World Health Organisation estimates that by applying existing knowledge about prevention and treatment, cancer incidence in 2020 could be reduced from twenty million to fifteen million and cancer deaths could be reduced from ten million to six million.' The

World Cancer Research Fund UK (www.wcrf-uk.org accessed December 2004) recommend the following six simple cancer prevention tips for men:

1. Choose a diet rich in a variety of plant-based foods. The suggestion is seven or more daily portions of cereals, pulses or legumes, such as beans, lentils, peas, roots and tubers, such as potatoes, nuts and seeds.
2. Eat plenty of vegetables and fruits — five or more portions per day. It is estimated that this could reduce cancer rates by more than 20%.
⌘ Beta-carotene is found in vegetables and fruits that are a deep yellow-orange in colour. Once eaten, it is converted into Vitamin A. Diets high in beta-carotene are thought to protect against lung cancer and possibly oesophageal, gastric and colon cancer.
⌘ Diets rich in vitamin C, found in many vegetables and fruits, are thought to protect against gastric cancer and possibly cancers of the mouth, pharynx, oesophagus, lung, pancreas and cervix.
⌘ Foods rich in vitamin E are thought to protect against lung and cervical cancers.
3. Maintain a healthy weight and be physically active. Sixty minutes of moderate exercise per day may be required to maintain a healthy weight in someone who is otherwise sedentary.
4. Don't drink alcohol, but if you must, drink it in moderation. Men should restrict their intake to fewer than two drinks per day and avoid excessive or binge drinking. Research by Ruano-Ravina *et al* (2004) suggests that since red wine contains tannins, which are antioxidants, and resveratrol, which inhibits tumours developing or spreading, drinking it may protect against cancer. However, the researchers stress that drinking red wine excessively would outweigh any beneficial effects.
5. Select foods low in fat and salt. Limit consumption of animal (saturated fats) and do not eat more than six grams (one heaped teaspoon) of salt a day.
6. Prepare and store foods safely. Some moulds and fungus on foods produce mycotoxins, substances that are implicated in promoting cancers.
7. Individuals who are not vegetarians are advised to moderate their intake of preserved meat (eg. sausages, salami, bacon, ham). It is suggested that preserved meat is associated with an increased risk of colon cancer, whereas fresh meat is not.
8. Never eat foods or drinks at a very hot (scalding) temperature.
9. Do not smoke or use tobacco in any form.

By adopting these six tips, the risk of developing cancer could be reduced by 30–40%. This means preventing 100,000 cases of cancer in the UK and three to four million worldwide, every year.

Lung cancer

The numbers of new cases of lung cancer in any given year reflect the past smoking habits of men and women. In men, lung cancer rates have been decreasing since the 1970s, about 20 years after the decline in the numbers of men smoking.

Cancer Research UK (2002a)

On average in the UK, ninety-two people die from lung cancer every day — one person every fifteen minutes.

Cancer Research UK (2002b)

Most lung cancers start in the lining of the bronchi, but they can also begin in other areas such as the trachea, bronchioles or alveoli and can take years to develop. Lung cancer is a life-threatening disease because it often spreads to other parts of the body (metastasis) before it is found (American Cancer Society www.cancer.org accessed February 2005).

Lung cancer is the most common cancer occurring in Europe, and it accounts for nearly 25% of all new cancer cases in European men (307,000). The highest incidence of lung cancer in men is now found in eastern European countries such as Hungary, Poland, Russia, Czech Republic and Slovakia (Bray *et al*, 2001). Of the countries making up the EU, Greece has the highest rate of smoking in men and Sweden the lowest (Cancer Research UK, 2002a). In 2000, in the UK, about 34,000 people died from lung cancer (Hecht, 2002).

In their fact sheet on smoking and respiratory disease, ASH (2002) states that in 1999, 29,406 people in England and Wales died of lung cancer. In Scotland, more than 26,000 people are diagnosed as having lung cancer each year, and 15,000 die from it each year. Lung cancer is now the leading cause of premature death among Scots, having overtaken CHD (Scottish Executive 2001b). 'For lung cancer, the incidence rates among people living in the most deprived areas of Scotland are three times higher than the rates in the least deprived areas' (Scottish Executive, 2001: 26).

Cancer Research UK (2004) provides the following information (*Table 3.1*) on the number of new cases of lung cancer in the UK in 2001.

Table 3.1: New cases of lung cancer in the UK in 2001					
	England	**Wales**	**Scotland**	**N. Ireland**	**UK**
Males	18,577	1181	2402	544	22,704
Females	11,963	758	1723	302	14,744
Total	30,540	1937	4125	846	37,448

It is evident that there is a downward trend in male mortality from lung cancer in the UK, which reflects the fall in tobacco consumption in the male population. However, despite this, lung cancer remains the leading cause of male deaths from cancer (Cancer Research UK, 2004).

Box 3.3: Key facts about lung cancer

- ⌘ Lung cancer is the second most commonly diagnosed cancer in men.
- ⌘ There are roughly three male cases of lung cancer for every two female cases.
- ⌘ The trends in incidence and mortality for men and women are very different, which is entirely due to past smoking habits.
- ⌘ Lung cancer accounts for 25% of all male cancer deaths.
- ⌘ Survival rates of patients with lung cancer are very poor. The median survival in the UK is about five months
- ⌘ Of all the cancers, only the liver, pancreatic and cancer of the pleura have worse five-year survival rates in England & Wales.

Source: Cancer Research UK (2004); Melling *et al* (2002).

Causes of lung cancer

Fifty years ago, the work of professors Richard Doll and Austin Bradford-Hill first proved the link between smoking and lung cancer.

Cancer Research UK (2002b)

According to Hecht (2002), cigarette smoking causes roughly 87% of lung cancer cases. It is also implicated in causing 30% of all cancer deaths in the more developed countries in the world. The ASH fact sheet on smoking and respiratory disease reports of a study of male British doctors that identified deaths from lung cancer in smokers and non-smokers. In the fact sheet, they report several findings, summarised in *Table 3.2.*

Table 3.2: Deaths from lung cancer in smokers and non-smokers

Number of cigarettes smoked per day	Annual death rate per 100,000 men
0	10
1–14	78 (8 times that of non-smokers)
15–25	127 (13 times that of non-smokers)
25 or more	251 (25 times that of non-smokers)

Box 3.4: Key facts about smoking

- About twelve million adults in the UK smoke cigarettes: 28% of men and 24% of women.
- Adult smoking rates vary across the UK: East of England, 25% of people; North-West of England, 30%; Scotland, 31%; and 27% in Wales.
- Smoking is highest amongst those aged twenty to twenty-four: 38%of men and 34% of women in this age-group smoke.
- More than 80% of smokers start their habit as teenagers.
- In the UK, about 450 children start smoking every day.
- Eighteen per cent of boys and 26% of girls are regular smokers, despite the fact that it is illegal to sell cigarettes to those under the age of sixteen.
- Twenty per cent of men in professional occupations smoke compared with 34% in routine and manual occupations.
- Every year, around 114,000 smokers in the UK die as a result of their habit.
- Smoking causes about 30% of all cancer deaths (including about 84% of lung cancer deaths); 17% of all heart disease; and at least 80% of deaths from bronchitis and emphysema.

Source: ASH (2005).

Second-hand smoke (also known as environmental tobacco smoke or passive smoking) is now widely accepted to be a cause of lung cancer, but the risk is far lower than that in smokers (Hecht, 2002). Just thirty minutes' exposure is enough to reduce coronary blood flow (ASH, 2004a). Smokers are twenty-two times more likely to die from lung cancer than are non-smokers, and smoking at an early age is associated with an increase risk (Khuder *et al*, 1998). Hole

(2004) states that about 1000 deaths every year in Scotland can be attributed to second-hand smoke with forty-four of these related to lung cancer, whilst the majority are related to ischaemic heart disease (n=395), stroke (n=335) and respiratory diseases other than lung cancer (n=91).

Zmuda and Barton (2000: 1) report that 'according to research… smoking marijuana may pose a significant lung cancer risk. Commenting on the cancer danger of marijuana as compared with regular cigarettes, the University of California at Los Angeles researchers said the tar inhaled in marijuana smoke contains higher concentrations of carcinogenic hydrocarbons, including benzapyrene, a key factor in lung cancer. And the National Institutes of Health point out: marijuana smoke deposits four times as much tar in the respiratory tract asa comparable amount of tobacco, thus increasing exposure to carcinogens.' Apart from cigarette smoking, other risk factors for lung cancer include passive smoking, asbestos, radon, chemical carcinogens, previous chronic inflammatory lung disease and genetic predisposition (Virtamo, 1999).

Why do some smokers develop lung cancer while others can smoke all their lives and never develop it? 'Less than 20% of smokers get lung cancer. At present, we cannot predict which smoker is susceptible… Factors which could influence individual susceptibility to lung cancer in smokers include the extent of carcinogen uptake, metabolic activation and detoxification and DNA repair ability…' (Hecht, 2002: 464).

Risk factors for lung cancer

⌘ Smoking, since smoke inhalation damages the normal cleansing processes by which the lung protects itself. Smoking causes the cilia to be less effective. Cancer-producing agents (carcinogens) in the cigarette smoke will remain trapped in the airways. These chemicals can lead to the alteration of normal lung cells and, eventually, cancer. One in two smokers dies prematurely; of these, nearly one in four will die of lung cancer.

⌘ The more someone smokes, the more likely they are to develop lung cancer.

⌘ The risk of dying from lung cancer increases with the number of cigarettes smoked per day, although the duration of smoking is the strongest determinant.

⌘ Filtered and low-tar cigarettes only reduce risk slightly.

⌘ Fifteen years after an individual has stopped smoking, their risk of developing lung cancer is the same as that of a non-smoker.

⌘ Pipe and cigar smokers are much more likely to develop lung cancer than non-smokers (although their risk is lower than cigarette smokers).

⌘ Passive smokers are put at risk in the same way as smokers, albeit to a lesser extent, from inhalation of smoke.

⌘ People who are exposed to radon gas, a radioactive gas occurring naturally in soil and rock, found in particular parts of the country, such as areas of Cornwall and Devon.

⌘ People who are exposed to asbestos, a material used until the 1970s in industries such as ship-building, asbestos mining and construction.

⌘ People who are exposed to other chemicals, such as arsenic, vinyl chloride, nickel chromate, cola and coal-tar products, mustard gas and chloromethyl ethers.

⌘ Those who consume a poor diet — one low in vegetables and fruits, but high in total fat, saturated fat and alcohol.

⌘ Scientists have recently shown that smoking marijuana and crack-cocaine also increases a person's risk of developing lung cancer (ALCASE, 1999).

Sources: World Cancer Research Fund, 'Reducing your risk of lung cancer': www.wcrf-uk.org.uk/publications/; Cancer Research UK, 'Risks and Causes of Lung Cancer': www.cancerhelp.org.uk (accessed January 2003); ASH (2004) Fact Sheet 4 'Smoking and Cancer': www.ash.org.uk/html/factsheets/pdfs/fact04.pdf (accessed January 2005).

Young people and smoking

ASH (2002: 2) states that 'children become aware of cigarettes at an early age. Three out of four children are aware of cigarettes before they reach the age of five, whether the parents smoke or not. By the age of eleven, one-third of children, and by sixteen years, two-thirds of children, have experimented with smoking. In Great Britain, about 450 children start smoking every day... The proportion of regular smokers increases sharply with age: 1% of eleven-year-olds smoke regularly, compared with 22% of fifteen-year-olds... Children are three times more likely to smoke if both their parents smoke and parents' approval or disapproval of the habit is also a significant factor... Children who smoke are two to six times more susceptible to coughs, increased phlegm, wheeziness and shortness of breath than those who do not smoke. One study revealed that children who smoke are three times more likely to have time off school.'

Levi (1999: 1914) calls for 'a comprehensive European tobacco policy... to reduce the health consequences of tobacco smoking, and this should be targeted via a variety of actions aimed at stopping young people starting smoking and to help smokers to quit.' This is particularly important, since it is evident that whilst there has been a decline in smoking among British adults, the same cannot be said of young people (MacFadyen *et al*, 2003). MacFadyen *et al* argue that the reason for this is that young people perceive smoking as something that enhances their self image.

MacFadyen *et al* (2003) continue in their exploration of why young people smoke by pointing out that adolescents think that smoking signals to others their adult status, coupled with the belief that they will be able to stop smoking at any time because they are in control. 'However, social smoking may be more risky than these young people believed. Recent research with younger adolescents has found that the first symptoms of nicotine dependence can appear within weeks or even days of occasional use, often before the onset of daily smoking' (MacFadyen *et al*, 2003: 497).

Sutherland and Shepherd (2001) conducted a large survey of 4516 English schoolchildren between the ages of eleven and sixteen. They found that individuals who perceived they had low educational achievement were twice as likely to smoke; 1.3 times more likely to drink alcohol; and 2.5 times more likely to use illegal drugs than those who perceived they had done well educationally. They also noted that adolescents who did not have any religious convictions were 2.1 times more likely to smoke cigarettes; 2.8 times more likely to drink alcohol; and 2.5 times more likely to use illicit drugs than their counterparts who did have religious convictions.

Once young people become weekly smokers, it is unlikely that they will stop, despite several attempts to do so. Stopping smoking successfully is dependent on the extent of smoking among their peers (Paavola *et al*, 2001). Stimuli to give up smoking include being asked to by their boyfriend or girlfriend, or doing so for health or financial reasons. Paavola *et al* (2001) state that smoking cessation was more common if their best friend was a non-smoker. In a cross-sectional survey of 17,287 high-school students in the USA, Wakefield *et al* (2000) found that the transition of teenagers through the stages of taking up smoking was reduced by bans on anyone smoking at home and also by restrictions on home smoking. Bans in public places also reduced smoking uptake, but had less effect than home bans. Smoking bans in schools had little effect unless strongly enforced.

Signs and symptoms of lung cancer

Chest signs/symptoms

- smoker's cough that persists or becomes intense
- persistent chest, shoulder or back pain
- increase in volume of, or change in colour of, sputum
- blood in sputum (haemoptysis)

- persistent hoarseness
- sudden onset of wheezing
- cough, even in non-smokers, that persists for more than two weeks
- repeated episodes of pneumonia or bronchitis

Other signs/symptoms

- fatigue
- loss of appetite
- headache, bone ache or aching joints
- bone fractures not related to accidental injury
- unexplained weight loss
- unsteady walk and occasional memory lapses
- neck and facial swelling

Source: World Cancer Research Fund, 'Reducing your risk of lung cancer'. ww.wcrf-uk.org.uk/publications/ (last accessed February 2005)

Prevention of lung cancer

The most effective way of preventing lung cancer is for people not to start smoking in the first place. For those who actually do smoke, stopping smoking is essential. In the UK, fourteen million people smoke (World Cancer Research Fund, www.wcrf-uk.org/publications/ accessed February 2005).

A recent study by Etter *et al* (2003) found that some individuals assume that smoking 'light' and 'ultra-light' cigarettes is less harmful than smoking regular cigarettes. This is not true. Etter *et al* state that because of this assumption, individuals switch from regular to light or ultra-light cigarettes, believing that they are reducing potential harm from smoking and use this concept as a rationale for delaying stopping smoking. Furthermore, Etter *et al* postulate that young people may start smoking light or ultra-light cigarettes, believing that they are not as harmful as regular cigarettes, and that if these individuals were aware of the true facts they may not start smoking at all.

So what are the facts about light and ultra-light cigarettes? 'Epidemiologic studies suggest that smoking low-tar cigarettes may even increase the risk of lung adenocarcinoma... low-tar cigarettes may cause different forms of lung cancer, but not necessarily fewer cases. Finally, smoking low-yield cigarettes does not reduce the risk of heart disease. 'Thus it is doubtful whether light cigarettes reduce the risk of disease or of becoming addicted to tobacco' (Etter *et al*, 2003: 93). As a result of their findings, Etter *et al* (2003: 96) state, 'to avoid misinterpretation of "light" or "ultra-light" labels, these labels should be abandoned and cigarette packs should indicate that there is no evidence that current lower yield cigarettes reduce the risk of cancer, heart attack, stroke and pulmonary disease compared to that of current regular cigarettes.'

Smoking cessation

Using a focus-group method with a sample of eight men, Wakefield *et al* (1998) investigated smoking and smoking cessation among men whose partners were pregnant. They found that the most pervasive issue among the men was that passive smoking had more to do with discomfort or annoyance to non-smokers than with health risks, and was the underlying reason why some men did not smoke in their home environment. The researchers concluded that men require more information about the risks of passive smoking in pregnancy. By increasing their knowledge-base of the potential health risks, Wakefield *et al* (1998) believe that this may motivate men to stop smoking and support their partner in stopping too. According to Spinks (2003), smokers who stop smoking before they reach the age of thirty-five have a life expectancy close to that of those who have never smoked.

After stopping smoking for:

- twenty minutes — blood pressure and pulse return to normal
- seventy-two hours — breathing is easier, energy levels increase
- three months — erections are harder and sperm count is higher
- twelve months — risk of a heart attack is half that of a smoker
- five years — risk of lung cancer is half that of a smoker

Source: Dr Rob Hicks www.bbc.co.uk/health/mens/life_smoking.shtml
(last accessed February 2005)

ASH (2004) has calculated the amount of money that could be saved by stopping smoking (*Table 3.3*).

Table 3.3: Money spent on smoking based on the cost of a packet of main-brand cigarettes in April 2003 (£4.48)					
Cigarettes per day	Years of smoking				
	1	5	10	20	50
5	£409	£2044	£4088	£8176	£20,440
10	£818	£4088	£8176	£16,352	£40,880
20	£1635	£8176	£16,352	£32,704	£81,760
40	£3270	£16,352	£32,704	£65,408	£163,520

Source: ASH (2002) Fact Sheet 24 'Stopping smoking', ASH's 15 tips: www.ash. org.uk/html/factsheets/pdfs/fact24.pdf (last accessed January 2005)

Box 3.5: Key facts about smoking cessation

✱ Less than half the smokers who wish to quit succeed in stopping permanently before they reach the age of sixty.

✱ Around 104,800 people set a quit date through smoking cessation services.

✱ At the four-week follow-up, around 53,500 people had successfullyquit (based on self-report), 51% of those setting a quit date.

✱ Of those setting a quit date, the majority (81%) were aged between eighteen and fifty-nine; 1% were under eighteen and 19% were over sixty.

✱ The majority of people received Nicotine Replacement Therapy (NRT) or Bupropion (Zyban). About 53% of people received NRT only; about 26% received Bupropion only; and about 2% received both NRT and Bupropion. NRT releases a steady dose of nicotine into the bloodstream, easing withdrawal symptoms. Zyban is a drug that suppresses the part of the brain that gives smokers a nicotine buzz. It also reduces cravings and withdrawal symptoms.

✱ £138 million has been allocated between 2003 and 2006 to ensure the continued expansion and development of NHS Stop Smoking Services.

Sources: DoH (2002a, 2004)

Bovet *et al* (2002) carried out a study with the aim of examining whether making smokers aware that they had actually developed atherosclerotic plaques in their peripheral arteries would improve smoking cessation. The development of atherosclerotic plaques in peripheral arteries is commonly referred to as 'hardening of the arteries'. A sample of 155 participants who were classified as regular smokers was randomly assigned into one of two groups: group A received high-resolution ultrasonography of their carotid and femoral arteries and counselling to give up smoking; and group B received counselling only. After six months, all participants had a telephone interview with a nurse who was blind to the baseline number of cigarettes smoked by the participants and to the participant's group assignment. Bovet *et al* (2002: 217) believe the results of their study 'strongly suggest that providing smokers with photographs of ultrasonic images demonstrating their own atherosclerotic lesions together with relevant explanation resulted in a higher quit rate at six months compared to providing counselling only (22% vs. 6%).'

Other factors thought to reduce the risk of developing lung cancer

A study by Moysich *et al* (2002) suggests that regular aspirin use may be associated with reduced risk of lung cancer. Epidemiological studies consistently demonstrate that consumption of vegetables decreases the risk of lung cancer (Hecht, 2002). Birkett (1999) reports that twenty-four out of twenty-five studies demonstrated that individuals with a high intake of fruit and vegetables had a significantly lower risk of developing lung cancer. In Birkett's study (1999: 218), which involved a secondary analysis of data derived from the Ontario Health Survey of 38,000 participants, it was found that smokers ate less fruit and vegetables than non-smokers. 'Smokers also eat a diet which provides more calories from fat and has higher amounts of cholesterol and smaller amounts of fibre and calcium than do non-smokers... a large proportion of smokers fail to eat enough fruit and fruit juice to meet the standards expected to reduce cancer risk. This is particularly true for heavy smokers. Regular smoking is a strong risk factor for cancer. If smokers also eat a diet low in fruit and vegetables, they are at even higher risk of cancer. A comprehensive cancer prevention for smokers should adopt a multifactorial approach and include dietary counselling with respect to increasing fruit and vegetable intake.'

It is important to note that smoking cessation is of the utmost importance in prevention of lung cancer because quitting smoking causes roughly a tenfold drop in risk. The estimated drop in risk of an increased intake of fruit and vegetables is about a twofold decrease (Virtamo, 1999).

Screening for lung cancer

Unlike other cancers, screening is not effective in early detection of lung cancer. This is because individuals do not present with the disease until the cancer is well advanced. Screening of individuals who are asymptomatic through chest x-rays and sputum cytology have not been successful (Virtamo, 1999). It is for this reason that lung cancer is known as the silent killer. 'Despite advances in treatment of lung cancer, the five-year survival for lung cancer is only 10–15%. Thus the only efficient way to reduce the burden from lung cancer is prevention' (Virtamo, 1999: 329).

Colorectal cancer

The term 'colorectal' refers to the lower end of the large intestine — that is, the colon (or large bowel) and the rectum. colorectal cancer is the second most common cancer in both men and women in Europe, and the third most common cancer in Britain (World Cancer Research Fund www.wcrf.org.uk accessed January 2005) and it's the fourth commonest form of cancer worldwide (Boyle and Langman, 2000). There are some 30,000 new cases each year distributed fairly evenly between the sexes (Bray *et al*, 2001) and usually occurs in later life between the ages sixty and seventy years. Colorectal cancer kills about 20,000 people in the UK every year (Scholefield, 2000).

Colon and rectal cancers are slow-growing and treatment is most effective when it is caught early. 'The cancer begins growing on the inner wall of the colon and continues to grow deeper into the wall until it spreads into the abdomen and lymph nodes... If treated before it moves through the wall of the bowel, a cure rate of 91.4% is possible' (Lantz *et al*, 2001: 193).

Box. 3.6: Key facts about colorectal cancer

* Since the late 1970s, male colorectal cancer rates have increased by nearly 21% to almost 57 per 100,000 in the late 1990s. Female rates have remained fairly stable.
* Colorectal cancer is the third most commonly diagnosed cancer in the UK after lung and breast.
* It is the second most common cause of cancer death after lung, accounting for over 10% of all cancer deaths.
* Each year, there are about 35,000 new cases of bowel cancer diagnosed in the UK.
* For males, bowel cancer is the third most common cancer after lung cancer and prostate cancer, accounting for 14% of all cancers diagnosed in men.

⌘ There are more cases of colon cancer than rectal cancer. Rectal cancer is more common in men than in women.
⌘ In 2002, there were 16,000 deaths from colorectal cancer in the UK.Mortality rates are higher in men than in women.
⌘ Since the late 1970s, male colorectal cancer rates have increased by nearly 21% to almost 57 per 100,000 in 2000. Female rates have remained fairly stable.
⌘ Five-year survival rates for men with bowel cancer have improved over the past thirty years. Men diagnosed with colon cancer in the early 1970s had a five-year survival rate of 22%; men diagnosed in the late 1990s had a five-year survival rate of 47%.

Source: Cancer Research UK (2004)

Causes of colorectal cancer

Cells lining the inside of the bowel are constantly dying and being replaced. A cancer can arise when this process of renewal goes wrong. These cells then grow to form a polyp. Most polyps are benign and cause no harm, but some progress into cancer. There are several risk factors:

⌘ More common in fifty-and-over age-group.
⌘ Diets that are high in fact and calories and low in fibre are believed to account for 80% of cases.
⌘ Individuals with familial adenomatous polyposis: a rare, inherited condition that causes hundreds of benign polyps to form in the colon and which, if left untreated, is almost certain to lead to colorectal cancer.
⌘ There's also a strong genetic element to the disease. Around 6% of people with bowel cancer have a family history of the disease. You will have a four-fold increased risk of developing bowel cancer if a close relative (parent, child, brother, sister) was diagnosed before the age of forty-five. However, if you have a close relative who was diagnosed after the age of sixty, you have the same risk of developing this cancer as the rest of the population.
⌘ If you have a sedentary lifestyle or suffer from inflammatory bowel disease (such as ulcerative colitis or Crohn's disease), you run an increased risk of developing bowel cancer.

Source: http://www.malehealth.co.uk/userpage1.cfm?item_id=116
(last accessed January 2005)

The main symptoms of colorectal cancer, according to the male health website (http://www.malehealth.co.uk/userpage1.cfm?item_id=116#bc-symptoms [accessed January 2005]), are:

⌘ A change in bowel habits, such as constipation or diarrhoea; changes in stool consistency; anything that is abnormal, or which lasts beyond two weeks.

⌘ Rectal bleeding, blood mixed in the stools, or dark stools. (It is a mistake to think that only dark blood is bad news — depending on where the cancer is, the blood can be bright red.)

⌘ The feeling of still having to go to the toilet, even after emptying the bowels.

⌘ Abdominal pain.

⌘ Unexplaind weight loss.

⌘ Poor appetite.

⌘ Anaemia (low red-blood-cell count).

⌘ A lump in the abdomen.

⌘ Tiredness.

However, these symptoms can appear for many other non-life-threatening bowel conditions.

Preventing colorectal cancer

Colorectal cancer is one type of cancer that can be prevented by adopting a healthy diet and lifestyle. It is estimated that only 30% of colorectal cancers are due to genetic factors, the remainder being related directly to diet. 'Scientists estimate that as many as 66–75% of cases of colorectal cancer could be avoided if we follow the type of diet and life style recommended by WCRF' (www.wcrf.org.uk last accessed January 2005).

Boyle and Langman (2000) and the World Cancer Research Fund offer the following points in how individuals can reduce their risk of colorectal cancer:

⌘ Increase intake of vegetables and fruits (eat five servings of fruits and vegetables each day); replace snacks such as chocolate, biscuits and crisps with an apple, orange, or other fruit or vegetable. It is believed that vegetables help prevent the formation of polyps on the inner walls of the colon and rectum.

⌘ Increase intake of fibre from foods such as potatoes, brown rice, beans, wholegrain bread and cereals. It is thought that because of their high fibre content, these foods move through the colon quickly, so any carcinogens that have been ingested have a reduced time in direct contact with the inner lining of the colon and rectum.

⌘ Reduce intake of calories (animal fats in particular); try to replace beef, lamb and pork with fish and poultry.

⌘ Increase physical activity through exercise of moderate intensity, such as brisk walking.

⌘ Participate in population-screening programmes; when these are not in place, strongly consider having a colonoscopy with polyp removal between the ages of fifty and fifty-nine.

⌘ Consult a doctor as soon as possible if a noticeable and unexplained change in bowel habit occurs — for example, blood is present in the stool; colicky pain occurs in the abdomen; or a sensation of incomplete evacuation after defecation recurs.

Sandhu *et al* (2001) conducted a meta-analysis to investigate the relationship between meat consumption and the risk of developing colorectal cancer. They found that there was an association between the consumption of red meat, particularly processed meat, and the risk of developing colorectal cancer. The advice of the World Cancer Research Fund is to limit intake of red meat to below 80g a day.

Being physically active is known to reduce the risk of developing colon cancer: 'physically active men and women experience around half the risk of their sedentary counterparts... physical activity reduces bowel transit time and thereby the duration of contact between faecal carcinogens and colonic mucosa...' (Batty and Thune, 2000: 1424).

Screening for colorectal cancer

It is possible to develop colorectal cancer without developing any of the above symptoms. Individuals who have a strong family history of colorectal cancer should have regular screening tests, which are normally carried out every three to five years. Examples of screening tests include barium enemas and colonoscopy. However, a non-invasive form of screening — the faecal occult blood test — can be effective in detecting colorectal cancer. These tests detect haematin from partially digested blood in the faeces (Scholefield, 2000).

'Two major European trials have been completed recently, showing that population screening based on testing of faeces for the presence of occult blood is effective in reducing mortality from colorectal cancer. The UK trial showed that the test was able to detect some asymptomatic, early-stage carcinomas and pre-malignant adenomas. Results of this trial point to a 15% reduction in mortality' (www.cancerbacup.org.uk/reports/cs/cs8.htm, January 2005).

According to Scholefield (2000), 'their [faecal occult blood tests] overall sensitivity for colorectal neoplasia is only 50–60%, though their specificity is high. In screening studies of faecal occult blood tests, individuals are invited to take two samples from each of three consecutive stools. Compliance is around

50–60%, but with population education this might be improved. Individuals with more than four out of six positive tests (about 2% of participants) need colonoscopy... The disadvantage of screening with faecal occult blood is its relatively low sensitivity — a third to a half of cancers will be missed on each round of screening. The Nottingham data suggest that screening every two years detects only 72% of cancers. This could be improved by testing annually and using more sensitive immunologically based faecal occult blood tests' (Scholefield, 2000: 1005).

Genetic testing for colorectal cancer is not widely available, but if an individual has three relatives with colorectal cancer (one aged under fifty) in two generations, it may be possible to identify the faulty or altered gene. Cancer BACUP (2003) is a good resource for reading more about genetic consultation and genetic counselling (http://www.cancerbacup.org.uk/Aboutcancer/Genetics/Cancergenetics/Geneticconsultationgeneticcounselling, January 2005).

Prostate cancer

Every year, around 19,000 men are diagnosed with prostate cancer in England and Wales. Around 8,500 men die from it.

NHSE (2000: 3)

Box 3.7: Key facts about prostate cancer

⌘ Causes of prostate cancer are unknown.
⌘ At least one in thirteen men in the UK will develop prostate cancer during their lifetime.
⌘ Around 27,000 new cases of prostate cancer are diagnosed in the UK each year. In 2000, prostate cancer claimed nearly 9,300 lives in the UK.
⌘ The highest rate of prostate cancer in the world is in men of African descent, and the lowest rates are in Far Eastern and Asian men.
⌘ It rarely affects men under the age of fifty.
⌘ Almost 90% of cases occur in men over the age of sixty-five.
⌘ If diagnosed early, the prognosis is good.
⌘ The incidence of prostate cancer has increased by more than 30% since 1993.

Sources: Institute of Cancer Research (2005); Cancer Research UK (2002c);
World Cancer Research Fund (2000)

> *Despite the scale of the problem, there is still a large degree of*
> *ignorance about prostate cancer within the male population: six out*
> *of ten men are unable to identify the early warning signs of prostate*
> *cancer, and only one in eight know what the prostate gland does.*

prostate cancer is the second most common cancer in men. There are about 85,000 new cases and between 35,000 and 40,000 deaths per year. It has been predicted that prostate cancer will overtake lung cancer in men by 2006 (www. icr.ac.uk/everyman/about/prostate.html accessed January 2005). In England and Wales, there are 17,000 new cases diagnosed and over 8,500 deaths per year (Neal and Donovan, 2000; Neal *et al*, 2000). Typically, those who die do so between four and five years after the diagnosis (NHSE, 2000). It is estimated that the number of men with prostate cancer will rise as the elderly population rises. 'The prevalence of diagnosed prostate cancer will increase from about 48,531 to 64,814 and thus, the total number of consultations with GPs will increase from 189,271 to 252,775' (Chamberlain *et al*, 1997: iii). The World Cancer Research Fund states that one in every thirteen British men will develop prostate cancer at some point during their lifetime. It rarely develops in men under forty years of age and most commonly occurs in men over sixty-five. Irish-born men have twice the incidence of prostate cancer than all other men (Lees and Papadopoulos, 2000).

Prostate cancer can be one of two types: first, the slow-growing, non-fatal type; second, the asymptomic, aggressive, fast-growing type, whereby the tumour metastasises quickly, often before any symptoms are noticed. In the slow-growing type, the individual may not experience any problems at all during their lifetime (NHSE, 2000). It is for this reason that prostate cancer is referred to as the most mysterious of all cancers, as it is often impossible to distinguish between slow-growing and fast-growing tumours (NHSE, 2000).

Causes of prostate cancer

The actual cause of prostate cancer is as yet unknown (NHSE, 2000). There is thought to be a genetic link because men who have first-degree relatives with prostate cancer have an increased risk of the disease. Those men whose relatives were diagnosed with the disease before the age of fifty-five are at particular risk. Neal *et al* (2000) state that a forty-year-old man with a close relative (father, uncle, brother) with the disease will have a 30–40% lifetime risk of developing clinically significant disease. One close relative with the disease, or who had had the disease, increases the risk twofold. Having two close relatives with a history of the disease increases the risk fourfold (NHSE, 2000). However, Chamberlain *et al* (1997) state that fewer than 10% of all prostate cancer cases appear to be inherited.

It is also suggested that a diet high in animal fats and milk products may be a risk factor, whilst a diet that is rich in green vegetables may be protective (Everyman website: http://www.icr.ac.uk/everyman/prostate_faq.html accessed January 2005). Moreover, a diet containing moderate or high amounts of fatty fish such as salmon, herring and mackerel may be a protective factor. A Swedish study of 6,200 men discovered that men who did not eat fish were two to three times more likely to develop prostate cancer (male health forum).

Certain ethnic groups have a higher incidence of prostate cancer than others. African-Caribbean or African-American men are more likely to develop prostate cancer, whereas Asian men have a lower risk (CancerBacup: www.cancerbacup.org.uk/Cancertype/Prostate/Causesdiagnosis/Symptoms, accessed January 2005).

Symptoms of prostate cancer

The slow-growing tumours commonly cause men few problems; indeed, many men may have prostate cancer and be totally unaware of it. The prognosis of prostate cancer is such that men often die with prostate cancer rather from it. However, up to 1% of men under fifty will develop invasive prostate cancer in the subsequent ten years (www.york.ac.uk).

Symptoms of prostate cancer do not present until the later stages of the disease. When they do occur, they present as:

- difficulty in passing urine
- hesitancy before urine begins to flow
- passing urine more frequently than usual, especially at night
- pain on passing urine
- blood in the urine, but this is not common
- pain in the bones (if the cancer has spread to the bones)

Source: www.cancerbacup.org.uk/Cancertype/Prostate/Causes
diagnosis/Symptoms (accessed January 2005)

Screening for prostate cancer

Screening is a process by which asymptomatic individuals are tested to determine whether they are likely to have a certain disease. Screening aims to detect and treat a disease at an earlier stage than if it was detected after symptoms occurred, and in this way improves the prognosis. As yet, there is no evidence that prostate screening reduces mortality from prostate cancer.

Screening involves a Prostate Specific Antigen (PSA) test. PSA is produced naturally and specifically by the prostate gland, but not specifically by prostate cancer. The amount of PSA in the bloodstream is increased when the membranes within the prostatic ducts are damaged. The latter fact makes the blood test controversial, as a raised PSA does not necessarily indicate the presence of prostate cancer. Indeed, two out of three men with a raised PSA do not have prostate cancer; furthermore, men with prostate cancer may not have a raised PSA (www.cancerhelp.org.uk, accessed January 2005).

In the UK, there is no national prostate cancer screening programme because there is no evidence that such a programme would bring more benefit than harm. The NHS Cancer Screening Programmes therefore advocate the use of a Prostate Cancer Risk Management programme, which is based on providing men with information so that they can make an informed choice as to whether to take a PSA test or not. (There is an information sheet at www.cancerscreening. nhs.uk/prostate/prostate-patient-info-sheet.pdf, accessed January 2005.)

Reducing the risk of prostate cancer

According to the World Cancer Research Fund (2000), scientific evidence is beginning to accumulate to suggest that a healthy diet and lifestyle may help reduce the risk of prostate cancer. A possible protective factor is antioxidants, which are thought to prevent the cell damage caused by free radicals. Examples of antioxidants are Vitamin C, Vitamin E and Selenium, which are found in many fruits and vegetables. Therefore, diets that are high in fruit and vegetables are associated with a lower prostate cancer risk, while those which have a high animal (saturated) fat content are linked to an increase risk of prostate cancer (World Cancer Research Fund 2000). Neergaard (2002) reports the outcome of one study that found that lycopene, which is the antioxidant that makes tomatoes red, lowered prostate cancer by 35%.

Testicular cancer

Testicular cancer is uncommon and accounts for only 1% of all male cancers worldwide. However, it is one of the commonest malignancies in young men (Aareleid *et al*, 1998). It is most commonly seen in men between the ages of twenty and forty-four, but can develop as early as fifteen years of age (www. icr.ac.uk, January 2005). The peak incidence is said to be between twenty-five and thirty-five years of age (Dearnaley, 2001). It is suggested that one in 500 men will develop testicular cancer, and nearly 2000 men are diagnosed with it every year in the UK (www.icr.ac.uk, January 2005; www.cancerhelp.org.uk, last accessed January 2005).

The incidence of testicular cancer is rising in the Western male population. England, Germany, France and Italy are amongst the leading nations for testicular cancer. The incidence of testicular cancer in the UK has risen by 70% in the past twenty years for as yet unknown reasons (www.health_icr.ac.uk, accessed January 2005). Irvine (2000) notes that in the west of Scotland, the number of cases of testicular cancer more than doubled between 1960 and 1990. In the UK, the lifetime risk of developing testicular cancer is one in 259 (www. cancerresearch.org.uk, last accessed January 2005).

The cause of testicular cancer is yet unknown but it is speculated that it may be due to genetic and environmental factors (Dearnaley *et al*, 2001). There is a strong genetic component: close relatives (brothers, fathers, sons) of individuals with testicular cancer have ten times increased risk of developing the disease (www.icr.ac.uk, accessed January 2005). In February 2000, the Institute of Cancer Research found a testicular cancer gene abnormality called TGCT1, which stands for Testicular Germ Cell Tumour 1. The abnormal gene was found on the X chromosome, so it is inherited from the mother rather than the father. The researchers believe that there may be another three abnormal genes yet to be discovered and they estimate that one in five testicular cancers could be due to inheriting faulty genes (www.cancerhelp.org.uk, accessed January 2005).

Dearnaley *et al* (2001) note that because of the age distribution of testicular cancer, it is likely than some sort of initiating event occurs prenatally, and that the tumour develops from adolescence. One plausible theory, not yet fully proven, is that testicular tissues are damaged while male foetuses are still developing, possibly as a result of their mothers' exposure to environmental pollutants that are chemically similar to the female hormone, oestrogen. It may be that male foetuses are being over-exposed to oestrogen and that, as a result, some develop a range of problems with their reproductive systems.

Although the cause of testicular cancer is unknown, there are a number of identified risk factors, one of which is undescended testicles. Testicles are formed in the abdomen of male fetuses and move down into the scrotum at birth or will descend within the first year of life. If they do not move down into the scrotal sac after this time, they are termed 'undescended'. It is known that men who have undescended testicles have a ten times increased risk of developing testicular cancer (www.cancerhelp.org.uk). Carrying out corrective surgery in boys with undescended testicle(s) before the age of six years can dramatically reduce the risk (Moore and Topping, 1999), but these individuals still have a higher risk than men without undescended testicles (www.cancerhelp.org.uk, January 2005). There is a small risk of developing testicular cancer if a man has fertility problems. It used to be thought that there was a connection between having a vasectomy and developing testicular cancer, but this was found to be false (www.cancerhelp.org.uk).

Signs and symptoms of testicular cancer

The common presentation of testicular cancer is a painless lump in one testicle (it rarely involves both testicles). The painless lump or swelling is often discovered by chance by the man or his partner (Dearnaley *et al*, 2002). In the early stages, there are no symptoms. When symptoms do appear, they include enlarged testicle; a feeling of heaviness in the testicle or groin; blood or fluid that accumulates suddenly in the scrotum; or a sore that doesn't heal (www.icr.ac.uk; www.cancerhelp.org.uk, accessed January 2005). Just as most lumps in the female breast are not cancerous, the same applies to lumps found in the testicles. Fewer than 40% of lumps found in the testicles turn out to be cancerous (www.cancerhelp.org.uk, accessed January 2005).

The prognosis of testicular cancer is good if it is diagnosed early. Indeed, if discovered early, there is a 80–90% cure rate (www.icr.ac.uk, accessed January 2005). Due to advances in treatment, including combination chemotherapy and the introduction of cisplatin (Aareleid *et al*, 1998), even individuals who have tumours that have spread can gain an 80% cure rate. However, for those with large-volume tumours, the cure rate can be as low as 44% (Barling and Lehmann, 1999; www.icr.ac.uk, accessed January 2005).

Testicular self-examination

Since the prognosis is best if the disease is diagnosed early, it is imperative that men are aware of the signs and symptoms so they can take appropriate action. For this reason, testicular self-examination (TSE) (see *Box 3.8*) is recommended once a month from the age of puberty until forty years of age (Barling and Lehmann, 1999). However, research indicates that, in general, men do not perform TSE despite its value, nor do they have adequate knowledge of testicular cancer or TSE (Lantz *et al*, 2001).

Barling and Lehmann (1999) carried out a quantitative survey of a convenience sample of 101 male university students between the ages of eighteen and twenty-five. The mean age was 22.9 years. The results confirmed previous findings that most men are uninformed or misinformed about testicular cancer and TSE. They expressed particular concern regarding one of their findings — that the overwhelming majority of the respondents did not know that testicular cancer was most likely to occur in their age-group.

Also in 1999, Moore and Topping carried out a quantitative descriptive survey with a purposive convenience sample of 203 full-time male undergraduate and postgraduate students. The sample was between the ages of eighteen and forty-five with a mean age of 22.5 years. Some 192 students completed questionnaires. The findings were similar to those of Barling and Lehmann (1999). In terms of identifying the most at-risk age group, 45.8% (n=88) responded correctly, whilst 42.2% (n=81) didn't know which group was most at risk. Moore and Topping (1999) report that those who were aware of the correct group were more likely to perform TSE once a month. When asked about TSE, 32.2% (n=63) said they had been informed about it and forty-three of these men practised it. Their knowledge of it arose from a variety of sources: newspaper or magazine (14%; n=22); pamphlet (13%; n=21); a nurse or doctor (11%; n=18); and from a friend (3%; n=5).

A Dutch survey by Lechner *et al* (2002) using 274 young men between the ages of fifteen and nineteen attending senior high school revealed more alarming findings: 74% of the sample had never heard of testicular cancer; only 3% had heard of TSE; and only 2% reported regularly practising it. White (2001) reports that in the UK, the Orchid Cancer Appeal is distributing videos to schools with the aim of spreading the message of the importance of TSE in the fifteen to sixteen year-old age groups. Moreover, White (2001) believes that healthcare professionals should consciously and regularly ask men between the ages twenty and thirty-five whether they are aware of the importance of TSE and check whether they know how to do it (*Box 3.8*).

Testicular cancer often occurs at an age when good health is taken for granted, so it is important that there is increased public education and awareness to help individuals avoid unnecessary delays in presentation, which may have a direct bearing on their survival (Dearnaley, 2001). A study done by Jones and Appleyard (1989) found that, on average, men waited fourteen weeks from the onset of symptoms to seeking a consultation with a doctor.

Other diseases predominantly affecting men

Prostate disease

Prostate problems are the main health problems for men over forty years of age (Pateman and Johnson, 2002; Summer *et al*, 2002). The prostate gland is the size of a walnut, surrounds the urethra, and is situated below the bladder and in front of the rectum. It produces a thick fluid — prostate fluid — which forms part of semen. Prostate fluid provides semen with its characteristic milky colour and makes up about one third of the entire ejaculate volume (Prostate Cancer Charity, 2003a).

A Mori poll carried out in 2001, on behalf of the Prostate Cancer Charity, showed that men's knowledge of their prostate was poor. Only 12% of men in the poll knew the function of the prostate gland, and 20% wrongly believed it to be situated in the testes. In new-born boys, the prostate is about the size of a pea and grows very slowly until puberty when there is a dramatic growth spurt as it doubles in size (www.malehealth.co.uk/userpage1.cfm?item_id=128, accessed January 2005).

It remains common for men to believe that urinary-tract symptoms are an inevitable consequence of ageing, as opposed to underlying disease. The Men's Health Forum note that there have been no national health promotion campaigns and that both men and their families would benefit from comprehensive information surrounding diagnosis, symptoms, treatment, interventions and other men's experiences of the conditions. Benign Prostate Hyperplasia, for example, has major effects on the quality of men's lives, yet there is little public awareness of the condition.

Box 3.8: How to do a TSE (testicular self-examination)

1. Perform after a warm bath or shower, as the skin around the scrotum is relaxed and soft.
2. Do it regularly to become familiar with the normal size, shape and weight of the testicles.
3. Stand in front of a mirror and assess the size and shape of both testicles. It is common to have one slightly larger, or for one to hang lower.
4. Hold your scrotum in the palm of your hand. Place your fingers under the testicle and your thumb on top. You should be able to feel a soft,tender tube at the top and back of the testicle. This is the epididymis that carries and stores sperm.
5. Gently roll each testicle between the thumb and fingers. It should be smooth, with no lumps or swellings.
6. Compare one testicle with the other: they should both feel the same.
7. A lump is not necessarily maligant; it may well be benign. But all lumps should be checked by a doctor.

Changes to watch for:

- any hard lump on a testicle (size of a pea or can be larger)
- swelling, enlargement or increase in firmness of a testicle
- a feeling of heaviness in the scrotum
- pain or discomfort in a testicle or the scrotum
- a dull ache in the groin
- any unusual difference between one testicle and the other

Sources: www.icr.ac.uk; www.cancerhelp.org.uk (last accessed January 2005)

There are three diseases that can affect the prostate gland: prostatitis; benign prostate hyperplasia; and prostate cancer.

Prostatitis

Prostatitis is an uncomfortable or painful inflammation or infection of the prostate gland; it can be acute or chronic in nature. Acute prostatitis is normally caused by a bacterial infection, whilst chronic prostatitis is less likely to be caused by a bacterial infection (Prostate Cancer Charity, 2003b). The chronic form is said to affect 9–14% of men worldwide (men's health forum) and can be particularly debilitating, as it causes persistent pelvic pain.

Acute bacterial prostatitis is caused by the transmission of bacteria either from infected urine or from sexually transmitted disease. The most common offending organism is E. Coli. In the UK, acute prostatitis can affect one in five men and accounts for about 25% of all consultations with urologists (Summer *et al*, 2002). The disease most commonly affects males in the age group thirty to fifty years of age. It is most commonly caused by an inflammation of the prostate gland, which causes a number of symptoms such as dysuria (pain during micturition), pyrexia and pain in any part of the pelvic or genital region. Acute prostatitis is treated with antibiotics. Chronic prostatitis occurs when men have repeated attacks of prostatitis. This can occur because of difficulty in treating the original infection or stopping antibiotic therapy too soon (Prostate Cancer Charity, 2003b). According to the Men's Health Forum, there is evidence to suggest that prostatitis is linked to psychological and work-related stress, and premature ejaculation.

Benign prostate hyperplasia (BPH)

Benign prostate hyperplasia (BPH) is a non-cancerous enlargement of the prostate. It is one of the commonest diseases to affect men over forty years of age and almost 50% of men over sixty-five suffer from problems caused by an enlarged prostate (Kirby, 2002). According to White (2001), BPH affects an estimated two million men in the UK and 40% of men in their seventies have clinical symptoms of BPH.

Roughly 500,000 men are diagnosed with BPH every year, but it is estimated that many more remain undiagnosed (2.5–3.5 million). The incidence of BPH increases with age. According to Kiviniemi and Suominen (1999), 25% of men aged fifty, over 40% of men aged sixty, and 80% of men aged over ninety, will have BPH.

Symptoms of BPH

BPH has several key symptoms (*Box 3.9*). Since the prostate surrounds the urethra, any enlargement will restrict the flow of urine from the bladder; it is this that produces the characteristic symptoms of stop-start urine flow, a feeling that the bladder is never fully emptied, and the frequent need to urinate. A particularly troublesome symptom is the need to pass urine several times during the night.

It has been noted that men with BPH are more likely to feel anxious and depressed than those without BPH. Having BPH can have a serious impact on men's social life, with many men unable to travel far from a toilet. The associated embarrassment is a factor in men delaying seeking medical attention. A Dutch study of almost 1000 randomly selected men aged fifty and over found that 20% had moderate to severe symptoms of BPH, but that the majority of these (60%) had not consulted their GP. Reasons given for the delay included embarrassment and lack of knowledge that their symptoms were due to an underlying disease.

Men's Health Forum have an online 'waterworks quiz' that aims to help men decide whether or not they need to seek medical advice (www.malehealth. co.uk/userpage1.cfm?item_id=128&pop=373, last accessed January 2005).

Box 3.9: Key symptoms of BPH

- dysuria — difficulty in passing urine
- a weak flow
- intermittency — a flow that starts and stops
- hesitancy — having to wait before you start to go
- frequency — having to urinate more often that previously
- urgency — finding it difficult to postpone urination
- nocturia — having to get up in the night to urinate

Source: www.malehealth.co.uk/userpage1.cfm?item_id=128&pop=373
(last accessed January 2005)

In terms of prevention, the following are suggested: increasing consumption of fruit and vegetables; introducing soya products into one's diet; and reducing one's intake of milk, red meat and saturated fat (www.malehealth.co.uk/ userpage1.cfm?item_id=128#bph-prevent, accessed January 2005).

Useful websites (all last accessed January 2005)

Action on Smoking and Health (ASH) provides information on the cost of smoking, both personally and to society — www.ash.org.uk

BBC's Health Website Cancer Guide — www.bbc.co.uk/health/cancer

CancerBACUP www.cancerbackup.org.uk – A patient support organisation that produces excellent literature. Cancer nurses staff their help and information line and it also offers cancer-counselling services

Cancer Link — www.njh.u-net.com/cancer.html

Cancer Research UK www.cancerresearchuk.org/ is a very informative website for patients

Colon Cancer Concern — www.coloncancer.org.uk

Cancer Counselling Trust — www.cctrust.org.uk

Database of individual patient experiences — contains interviews (as sound or video clips) with men who have had prostate cancer. www.dipex.org

Drug and medicines information — easy to use and free from medical jargon, it has patient information sheets that can be printed off: www.intelihealth.com

Imperial Cancer Research Fund — www.imperialcancer.co.uk

Institute of Cancer Research — www.icr.ac.uk

Macmillan Cancer Relief: www.macmillan.org.uk — contains information for patients and links to other organisations

Men's Health Forum is a charitable organisation that works to improve men's health by bringing together and working with the widest possible range of interested organisations and individuals — www.menshealthforum.org.uk

New Approaches to Cancer (ANAC) — www.anac.org.uk

NHS guide to health information on the internet — www.nhsdirect.nhs.uk

UK National Electronic Library for Health — covers all aspects of health, illness and treatments: www.nelh.nhs.uk

Orchid Cancer Appeal www.orchid-cancer.org.uk — contains information for men with testicular cancer

Patients Association — www.patients-association.com

Prostate Cancer Charity — www.prostate-cancer.org.uk

Prostate Help Association — www.pha.u-net.com

Prostate Research Campaign — www.prostate-research.org.uk

Sexual Dysfunction Association — www.sda.uk.net

Quitsmoking UK — an online community for quitting smokers by quitting smokers: www.quitsmokinguk.com, www.quitnet.org

World Cancer Research Fund — www.wcrf-uk.org

References

Aareleid T, Sant M, Hedelin G (1998) Improved survival for patients with testicular cancer in Europe since 1978. *Eur J Cancer* **34**(14): 2236–40

ALCASE (1999) *The Lung Cancer Manual*. Vancouver: Alliance for Lung Cancer Advocacy, Support and Education

ASH (2002) Fact Sheet No 3: Young People and Smoking. www.ash.org.uk/html/factsheets/html/fac03.html accessed January 2003

ASH (2004a) Fact Sheet 8 Second-hand Smoke. http://www.ash.org.uk/html/factsheets/pdfs/fact08.pdf (accessed January 2005)

ASH (2004b) Fact Sheet 7 Smoking, Sex and Reproduction. http://www.ash.org.uk/html/factsheets/pdfs/fact07.pdf (accessed January 2005)

ASH (2005) Basic Facts: One Smoking Statistics. http://www.ash.org.uk/html/factsheets/pdfs/basic01.pdf (accessed January 2005)

Barling NR, Lehmann M (1999) Young men's awareness, attitudes and practice of testicular self-examination: a Health Action Process Approach. *Psychol Health & Med* **4**(3): 255–63

Batty D, Thune I (2000) Does physical activity prevent cancer? *BMJ* **321**: 1424–5

Birkett NJ (1999) Intake of fruits and vegetables in smokers. *Public Health Nutr* **2**(2): 217–22

Bovet P, Perret MD, Cornuz J, Quilindo J, Paccaud F (2002) Improved smoking cessation in smokers given ultrasound photographs of their own atherosclerotic plaques. *Prev Med* **34**: 215–20

Boyle P, Langman JS (2000) ABC of colorectal cancer: epidemiology. *BMJ* **321**: 805–8

Bray F, Sankila R, Ferlay J, Parkin DM (2001) Estimates of cancer incidence and mortality in Europe in 1995. *Eur J Cancer* **38**(1): 99–166

Cancer BACUP (2001a) Familial risk and genetics in common cancers: bowel, breast and ovary. Cancer BACUP

Cancer BACUP (2001b) Current issues in the treatment of metastatic prostate cancer. Cancer BACUP

Cancer Research UK (2002a) Smoking and Cancer. September www.cancerresearchuk.org (accessed December 2004)

Cancer Research UK (2002b) Men's Cancer Factsheet May 2002. www.cancerresearchuk.org (accessed December 2004)

Cancer Research UK (2002c) Prostate Cancer Briefsheet June 2002. www.cancerresearchuk.org (accessed December 2004)

Cancer Research UK (2004) Large Bowel Cancer Factsheet April 2004. http://info.cancerresearchuk.org/images/publicationspdfs/factsheet_bowel_apr2004.pdf (accessed January 2005)

Cancer Research UK (2004) Lung Cancer Factsheet January 2004. www.cancerresearchuk.org accessed January 2005

Cancer Working Group (1999) Strategic Priorities in Cancer Research and Development. www.doh.gov.uk/research/documents/rd3/cancer_final_report.pdf (last accessed January 2005)

Carlisle D (2002) Cancer: the big picture. *Nurs Times* **98**(35): 22–3

Chamberlain J, Melia J, Moss S, Brown J (1997) The diagnosis, management, treatment and costs of prostate cancer in England & Wales. *Health Technol Assess* **1**(3): 1–68

Chapple A, Ziebland S, Shepperd S, Miller R, Herxheimer A, McPherson A (2002) Why men with prostate cancer want wider access to prostate specific antigen testing: a qualitative study. *BMJ* **325**: 737–40

Dearnaley DP, Huddart RA, Horwich A (2001) Managing testicular cancer. *BMJ* **322**: 1583–8

DoH (2002) Statistics on Smoking Cessation Services in Health Authorities: England, April to September 2001. www.doh.gov.uk/public/press14feb.htm (last accessed January 2005)

DH (2004) Statistical Bulletin: Statistics on NHS Stop Smoking Services in England, April 2003–March 2004. http://www.publications.doh.gov.uk/public/sb0418.pdf (last accessed January 2005)

Donovan JL, Frankel SJ, Neal DE, Hamdy FC (2001) Screening for prostate cancer in the UK. *BMJ* **323**: 763–4

Etter JF, Kozlowski LT, Perneger TV (2003) What smokers believe about light and ultralight cigarettes. *Prev Med* **36**: 92–98

Hecht SS (2002) Cigarette smoking and lung cancer: chemical mechanisms and approaches to prevention. *Lancet Oncol* **3**: 461–9

Hole DJ (2004) Passive Smoking and Associated Causes of Death in Adults in Scotland. Edinburgh: Health Education Board Scotland. www.hebs.com/researchcentre/pdf/moratalitystudy.pdf (last accessed January 2005)

Irvine DS (2000) Male reproductive health: cause for concern? *Andrologia* **32**: 195–208

Institute of Cancer Research (2005) Everyman: Action Against Male Cancer. http://www.icr.ac.uk/everyman/ (accessed January 2005)

Jones W, Appleyard I (1989) Early diagnosis of testicular cancer. *Practitioner* **233**: 509

Kiviniemi K, Suominen T (1999) 'Going to the bathroom four or five times a night...' seven men talk about their experiences of benign prostate hyperplasia and the perioperative period. *J Clin Nurs* **8**: 542–9

Khuder SA, Dayal HH, Mutgi AB, Willey JC, Dayal G (1998) Effect of cigarette smoking on major histological types of lung cancer in men. *Lung Cancer* **22**: 15–21

Korda M (1997) *Man to Man: Surviving Prostate Cancer*. London: Little, Brown & Company

Lantz JM, Fullerton JT, Harshburger RJ, Sadler GR (2001) Promoting screening and early detection of cancer in men. *Nurs Health Sci* **3**: 189–196

Lechner L, Oenema de Nooijer J (2002) Testicular self-examination (TSE) among Dutch young men aged 15–19: determinants of the intention to practice TSE. *Health Educ Res* **17**(1): 73–84

Lees S, Papadopoulos I (2000) Cancer and men from minority ethnic groups: an exploration of the literature. *Eur J Cancer Care (Engl)* **9**: 221–9

Leung LS, Yip AWC (1999) Sildenafil (Viagra) and erectile dysfunction. *Ann Coll Surg* **4**: 99–102

Levi F (1999) Cancer prevention: epidemiology and perspectives. *Eur J Cancer* **35**(14): 1912–24

Levine LA, Kloner RA (2000) Importance of asking questions about erectile dysfunction. *Am J Cardiol* **86**: 1210–13

Luck M, Bamford M, Williamson P (2000) *Men's Health: Perspectives, Diversity and Paradox.* Oxford: Blackwell Science

Lu-Yao G, Albertsen PC, Stanford JL, Stukel TA, Walker-Corkery ES, Barry MJ (2002) Natural experiment examining impact of aggressive screening and treatment on prostate cancer mortality in two fixed cohorts from Seattle area and Connecticut. *BMJ* **325**: 740–4

MacFadyen L, Amos A, Hastings G, Parkes E (2003) 'They look like my kind of people' — perceptions of smoking images in youth magazines. *Soc Sci Med* **56**: 491–9

Melling PP, Hatfield AC, Muers MF, Storer CJ, Round CE, Haward RA, Crawford SM (2002) Lung cancer referral patterns in the former Yorkshire region of the UK. *Br J Cancer* **86**: 36–42

Moore RA, Topping A (1999) Young men's knowledge of testicular cancer and testicular self-examination: a lost opportunity? *Eur J Cancer Care (Engl)* **8**: 137–42

Moysich KB, Menezes RJ, Ronsani A, Swede H, Reid ME, Cummings KM, Flakner KL, Loewen GM, Bepler G (2002) Regular aspirin use and lung cancer risk. **2**(31): 1–7

Neal DE, Donovan JL (2000) Prostate cancer: to screen or not to screen? *Lancet Oncol* **1**: 17–24

Neal DE, Leung HY, Powell PH, Hamdy FC, Donovan JL (2000) Unanswered questions in screening for prostate cancer. *Eur J Cancer* **36**: 1316–21

Neergaard L (2002) Nutrients are key to preventing cancer. http://www.intelihealth. com/IH/ihtIH/EMIHC000/333/8146/358666.html?d=dmtICNNews (last accessed December 2004)

NHSE (2000) *The NHS Prostate Cancer Programme.* London: NHS Executive

NHS Health Scotland & ASH Scotland (2004) Smoking Cessation Guidelines for Scotland. http://www.hebs.com/tobacco/professional/cessation_guidelines/ purpose.cfm (accessed January 2005)

Paavola M, Vartiainen E, Puska P (2001) Smoking cessation between teenage years and adulthood. *Health Educ Res* **16**(1): 49–57

Pateman B, Johnson M (2002) Men's lived experiences following transurethral prostatectomy for benign prostate hypertrophy. *J Adv Nurs* **31**(1): 51–8

Prostate Cancer Charity (2003a) What does the prostate do? www.prostate-cancer.org. uk/learn/prostate (last accessed January 2005)

Prostate Cancer Charity (2003b) Prostatitis. www.prostate-cancer.org.uk/learn/prostate (last accessed January 2005)

Prostate Cancer Charity (2003c) BPH www.prostate-cancer.org.uk/learn/prostate (last accessed January 2005)

Ruano-Ravina A, Figueiras A, Barros-Dios JM (2004) Type of wine and risk of lung cancer: a case control study in Spain. *Thorax* **59**: 981–5

Sandhu MS, Luben R, Khaw KT (2001) Systematic review of the prospective cohort studies on meat consumption and colorectal cancer risk: a metal-analytical approach. *Cancer Epidemiol Biomarkers Prev* **10**: 439–46

Scholefield JH (2000) ABC of colorectal cancer: screening. *BMJ* **321**: 1004–6

Scottish Executive (2001) Cancer in Scotland: Action for Change. Edinburgh: Scottish Executive. www.show.scot.nhs.uk/publications (accessed January 2005)

Spinks J (2003) Implementing NICE guidance: smoking cessation support. *Br J Health Care Manage* **9**(3): 104–7

Summer S, Dolan A, Thompson V, Hundt GL (2002) Prostate health awareness — promoting men's health in the workplace. *Men's Health J* **1**(5): 146–8

Sutherland I, Shepherd JP (2001) Social dimensions of adolescent substance use. *Addiction* **96**: 445–58

UK National Screening Committee (undated) Information sheet on screening for prostate cancer. www.cancerscreening.nhs.uk/prostate (accessed January 2005)

Virtamo J (1999) Vitamins and lung cancer. *Proc Nutr Soc* **58**: 329–33

Wakefield M, Reid Y, Roberts L, Mullins R, Gillies P (1998) Smoking and smoking cessation among men whose partners are pregnant: a qualitative study. *Soc Sci Med* **47**(5): 657–64

Wakefield MA, Chaloupka FJ, Kaufman NJ, Orleans CT, Barker DC, Ruel EE (2000) Effect of restrictions on smoking at home, at school, and in public places on teenage smoking: cross sectional study. *BMJ* **321**: 333–7

Wanless D (2002) *Securing Our Future Health: Taking a Long-term View. Final Report*. London: HM Treasury

White A (2001) *Report on the Scoping Study on Men's Health*. Edinburgh: HMSO

WHO (2002) *The European Health Report*. Copenhagen: WHO Europe

WHO (2003) Diet, Nutrition and the Prevention of Chronic Diseases. http://www. who.int/nut/documents/trs_916.pdf (accessed February 2005)

World Cancer Research Fund (1999) *Finding Out About Cancer. Information Series 2*. London: World Cancer Research Fund

World Cancer Research Fund (2000) *Reducing Your Risk of Prostate Cancer. Information Series 2*. London: World Cancer Research Fund

World Cancer Research Fund (UK) Reducing Your Risk of Colorectal Cancer. http://www.wcrf-uk.org/publications/leafletdetail.lasso?WCRFS=52299DE203011 2030EJtm3A8DD1B&SN=96 (last accessed February 2005)

World Cancer Research Fund (2002) *Diet and Health Recommendations for the Prevention of Cancer. Information Series 1*. London: World Cancer Research Fund

Zmuda R, Barton MK (2000) Lung Cancer. www.cancerpage.com/articles/print.asp?id =4&subarea=Prevention (accessed January 2005)

Chapter 4

Maintaining a healthy liver

The majority of the UK population drink; only 7% of men and 13% of women are non-drinkers.

Waller *et al* (2002: 5)

Alcohol is second only to tobacco as a cause of premature death amongst Britons.

World Cancer Research Fund UK (undated)

The number of alcohol-related deaths registered in England and Wales more than doubled between 1979 and 2000, from 2506 to 5543. Increases in death rates in younger age groups were especially large. The death rates for both men and women aged twenty-five to forty-four tripled between 1979 and 2000. The death rate for men aged forty-five to sixty-four exceeded that for men aged sixty-five and over.

Office of National Statistics (2003: 14)

Alcohol is an addictive drug that suppresses activity in the central nervous system. It promotes relaxation, eases anxiety, reduces inhibitions and has a deleterious effect on reactions, thought processes and co-ordination. It is also a carcinogen (World Cancer Research Fund UK, undated).

Alcohol is measured in units. One unit of alcohol is half a pint of beer (284ml); a single measure of spirits (25ml); or a standard glass of wine (125ml). The recommended level for men is fewer than twenty-two units per week and fewer than fifteen units a week for women (Guest and Varney, 2001). It is also recommended that individuals should have forty-eight hours free of alcohol following any episode where they drink over the daily recommended limits (Waller *et al*, 2002). Men are more likely than women to drink excessively (Menshealthforum): 27% of men drink more than the recommended limits and 36% of men aged sixteen to twenty-four drink excessively (White, 2001). The Institute of Alcohol Studies (2004a) states that the UK drinking culture reflects one of binge drinking, which is defined as drinking five or more standard drinks in one occasion. Moreover, British teenagers, along with their peers in Ireland and Denmark, are the heaviest drinkers in Europe.

Box 4.1: Key facts about alcohol consumption

⌘ Although it is difficult to ascertain the true extent of the rates of alcohol usage due to a tendency for self under-reporting, some 39% of men and 23% of women in the UK exceed the daily recommended limits (four and three, respectively).

⌘ Twenty-one per cent of men and 10% of women drink in binges.

⌘ It is estimated that there are around 1.9 million heavy drinkers (fifty units per week for men and thirty-six for women) in England.

⌘ It is estimated that about one in twenty adults in the UK are alcohol-dependent.

⌘ One in four male acute admissions to hospital are alcohol-related.

⌘ Alcohol is second only to tobacco as the main cause of preventable premature death in the UK.

⌘ It is estimated that healthcare costs related to alcohol misuse range from £1.4 to £1.6 billion.

⌘ In 2001, in England, it was estimated that there were 17 million working days lost due to alcohol misuse, leading to a total cost of absenteeism of £1.8 billion.

⌘ Moderate alcohol consumption can benefit health through improvements in social networking and reductions in stress and incidence rates of CHD.

⌘ Alcohol increases the risk of developing digestive disorders, cancer, liver cirrhosis, alcohol psychosis and is a major contributory factor in personal injuries.

⌘ Binge drinking can cause sudden cardiac death.

⌘ It is estimated that 6% of all road-traffic accidents and 16% of all road deaths in 2000 were caused by drivers exceeding the legal limit for alcohol.

⌘ Over the last thirty years, the numbers of men aged between forty-five and fifty-four who have liver cirrhosis had increased fourfold.

⌘ Cirrhosis of the liver is found in about 20% of all heavy drinkers.

⌘ It is estimated that there are between 5000 and 40,000 alcohol-related deaths in England and Wales every year.

Sources: Cabinet Office (2003); Alcohol Concern (2003); Royal College of Physicians

Definition of terms

Light/moderate drinker: A man who drinks fewer than twenty-one units a week and a woman who drinks fewer than fourteen units a week.

Heavy drinker: A man who drinks twenty-two to fifty units a week and a woman who drinks fifteen to thirty-five units a week.

Very heavy drinker: A man who drinks fifty-one or more units a week and a woman who drinks thirty-six or more units a week.

Source: Waller *et al* (2002: 26)

It is well known that having frequent episodes of heavy drinking or intoxication is a major predictor of alcohol-related problems. In all cultures, men drink more heavily than women (Makela and Mustonen, 2000). Worryingly, alcohol consumption in young people (eleven-fifteen age group) is increasing (Guest and Varney, 2001).

In their cross-sectional survey to assess the associations between drinking behaviour, gender and age, Makela and Mustonen (2000) used a sample of 3,446 Finnish people between the ages of fifteen and sixty-nine. They report that both genders gain social benefits from drinking. Men reported that drinking alcohol helped them to become more socially attractive, whilst women reported that alcohol helped them to share their feelings and personal problems.

According to the Department of Health (DoH) (2001a), 24% of school pupils in England had had an alcoholic drink in the previous week; 48% of fifteen-year-olds had drunk alcohol in the last week; and, according to estimates, the average consumption of alcohol in pupils rose from 5.3 units in 1990 to 10.4 units in 2000. Coleman and Hendry (1999) suggest that the increasing alcohol consumption in young adults is associated with the socialisation process into adulthood, with hangovers and other ill effects being accepted as part of a learning process.

Lintonen *et al* (2001) carried out a study with the aim of understanding early adolescent drinking within Finland. Their work was based on the Adolescent Health and Lifestyle Survey (n=2385) done in 1999 and aimed to identify characteristics related to heavy drinking in fourteen-year-olds. They found that all drinking seemed to be associated with a multitude of background and lifestyle factors. Being drunk was associated more among smokers than non-smokers. This was thought to be related either to being more likely to develop an addiction or to the role of alcohol and cigarettes in socialising with peers. Lintonen *et al* (2001: 165) concluded their paper with a portrait of a heavy drinker: 'If we were to identify a potential heavy drinker, we would look at the following factors. He/she is probably a smoker, living in a family with little parental control but with ample spending money to hand out to the adolescent. He/she may be biologically more mature than his/her peers and has started dating.'

Young people's drinking in UK

⌘ Hazardous drinking, defined as bringing the risk of physical or psychological harm, is found in 62% of men in the twenty to twenty-four years age-group.

⌘ The percentage of those drinking alcohol increases with age: 14% of twelve to thirteens; 33% of fourteen to fifteens; and 62% of sixteen to seventeens.

⌘ Ethnic minority teenagers are less likely to drink alcohol. One in twenty non-white twelve to seventeen year-olds are frequent drinkers, compared with one in four whites.

⌘ Despite the fact that it is illegal to buy alcohol under the age of eighteen, 63% of sixteen to seventeen year-olds and 10% of twelve to fifteen year-olds state that they have purchased alcohol in pubs, bars and nightclubs.

⌘ In Scotland, in the last twelve years, there has been a 60% increase in fifteen year-olds drinking alcohol, and more than a 100% rise in thirteen year-olds doing so.

⌘ Forty-two per cent of young men now exceed the recommended weekly alcohol limit, compared with 33% in 1997.

⌘ About 1000 young people a week sustain serious facial injuries as a result of drunken assaults. Some 18,000 young people each year are scarred for life.

⌘ UK teenagers are near the top of the international league for binge-drinking, drunkenness and alcohol-related problems.

⌘ Twenty-one per cent of teenagers who drink alcohol report having personal problems such as not doing so well at school; 22% report relationship problems; 15% report sexual problems (unwanted sexual experience or unprotected sex); and 12% report delinquency problems.

⌘ Since a teenager's tolerance of alcohol is lower than an adult's, they have a five times greater risk of having an accident when drink-driving compared with an adult drink-driving.

⌘ Young people who start drinking before they are fifteen are four times more likely to develop alcohol-dependence than those who start drinking at twenty-one.

⌘ Only 10% of adults who never drink have children who drink alcohol regularly, compared with 33% of adults who do drink three to four times a week.

⌘   Young people who come from single-parent families, lack parental control, truant from school, or have an elder sibling who uses a particular substance, are associated with an increased use of alcohol, tobacco smoking and cannabis smoking.

Source: Institute of Alcohol Studies (2005)

Male drinking patterns in the UK

- four million men binge-drink
- binge drinking accounts for 40% of all drinking occasions by men
- sixteen to twenty-four year-olds are the heaviest drinkers, with 50% of men drinking more than the recommended levels

Sources: Health Development Agency (2004); DoH (2003)

Drinking alcohol excessively is associated with socioeconomic factors such as poverty, disadvantage and lower social class. The highest proportion of men exceeding the recommended limits in 1998 was in Greater Glasgow, Scotland. Men in manual work are more likely to exceed eight units on their heaviest drinking day (Guest and Varney, 2001).

Alcohol misuse is common in jobs related to catering, brewing and distilling. High consumption of alcohol is perceived as the social norm in doctors, sailors and demolition workers. It is estimated that 33% of homeless people have alcohol problems (Ashworth and Gerada, 1997). Ashworth and Gerada (1997) state that British Afro-Caribbeans and South Asians have a lower than average consumption and lower admission rates for alcohol-related problems than white people. They also report that pockets of high consumption exist in Sikh men, who favour drinking spirits, and that about 20% of Chinese and Japanese people cannot drink alcohol because they have an inherited deficiency of acetaldehyde dehydrogenase, which is an enzyme necessary to metabolise alcohol. White (2001) states that South Asian men had an increasingly high use of drugs, alcohol and tobacco, which is reflected in an increase in liver disease in this population due to alcohol abuse.

Effects of alcohol on health and well-being

The health benefits of light or moderate drinking have been well publicised in relation to protection against heart disease for older

> *men... Unfortunately, regularly drinking above safe guidelines can take a terrific toll on the body as a whole and can contribute to a wide range of ill health, including coronary heart disease, strokes, impotence, cancer, liver cirrhosis, digestive problems and injury.*

> Alcohol Concern (undated)

When one considers the results of excessive alcohol intake, one of the commonest answers is the development of cirrhosis of the liver. Male deaths from liver disease and liver cirrhosis between 1988 and 1999 increased by 94% compared with a rise of 39% in women over the same time period (DoH, 2001b). The Chief Medical Officer's annual report in 2001 (DoH, 2001c) highlighted concerns regarding the increasing number of young men with chronic liver disease.

There is extensive and consistent evidence that alcohol also increases the risk of cancers developing in the upper aero-digestive tract — that is, anywhere alcohol comes in direct contact with the body: for example, mouth, pharynx, larynx and oesophagus (World Cancer Research Fund UK, undated). The World Cancer Research Fund UK (undated) state that other research shows that individuals who drink more than four to six alcoholic drinks daily are twice as likely to be at risk of developing colorectal cancers than non-drinkers. Alcohol Concern (undated) state that recent findings suggest that 80% of the aforementioned cancers could be avoided by abstaining from alcohol and tobacco. They also add gastritis, osteoporosis and sexual problems to the list of other health problems.

Alcohol is high in calories and therefore can lead to overweight or obesity. Alcohol is described as having empty calories in that despite being calorific it lacks vitamins, minerals and other essential nutrients found in food (World Cancer Research Fund UK undated).

If alcohol is used to relieve stress or worries, it can soon become a habit. Gradually, individuals may find that they have to increase their intake to achieve the desired effect and thus dependence occurs (Wise *et al*, 1995). Heavy drinking is harmful to health, as well as to the drinker's family and to society at large. As well as directly causing illnesses such as liver cirrhosis, alcohol contributes to certain cancers and stroke. Its misuse places families under stress, sometimes resulting in domestic violence, mental illness and family break-up, and it is a factor in many accidents (World Cancer Research Fund UK).

Alcohol consumption is associated with:

- 80% of suicides
- 50% of murders
- 80% of deaths from fire
- 40% of all road-traffic accidents
- 30% of fatal road-traffic accidents
- 15% of drownings

Alcohol consumption contributes to:

- One in three divorces
- One in three cases of child abuse
- 20–30% of all hospital admissions

Source: Ashworth and Gerada (1997)

Binge drinking

Binge drinking is a particular problem as the latest research indicates that the incidence of hypertension is approximately doubled in people who drink over six units per day.

Alcohol Concern (undated)

Binge drinking is defined as a man who regularly drinks ten or more units in a single session, or a woman who regularly drinks seven or more units in a single session.

Royal College of Physicians (2002)

The prevalence of binge drinking is highest among younger age groups. Only 25% of women and one in six men between the ages of eighteen and twenty-four report never drink-binging. Binge drinking has become so routine in this age group they find it difficult to explain why they do it, other than that it is part of their normal social scene (Institute of Alcohol Studies, 2004b). Binge drinking is strongly associated with:

- a deliberate intention to get drunk
- a need to escape from day-to-day pressures
- a need to feel confident, particularly with the opposite sex
- a desire to 'push the limits'
- conforming to peer-group pressure
- becoming over-confident and reckless and behaving in ways they would otherwise consider inappropriate or against their better judgement (for example, having unprotected sex or becoming aggressive)

Source: Engineer *et al* (2003)

Recognising when alcohol consumption becomes a problem

Ashworth and Gerada (1997) suggest five areas that may indicate a problem:

1. Amount of alcohol consumed in units.
2. Time of first alcoholic drink of the day.
3. Pattern of drinking — problem drinking is characterised by the establishment of an unvarying pattern of drinking.
4. Presence of withdrawal symptoms such as early-morning shakes or nausea.
5. Positive answers to the CAGE questionnaire (below).

The CAGE questionnaire consists of four questions:

1. Have you ever felt you should cut down on your drinking?
2. Have people annoyed you by criticising your drinking?
3. Have you ever felt bad or guilty about your drinking?
4. Have you ever had a drink first thing in the morning to steady your nerves or get rid of a hangover (eye-opener)?

Harm reduction

Waller *et al* (2002) outline the strategies and interventions that can be used to prevent alcohol misuse and alcohol-related harm. These include:

⌘ Use of taxation to raise the price of alcohol.
⌘ Restrictions on distribution outlets.
⌘ Restrictions on advertising.
⌘ Law enforcement (under-age purchasing of alcohol).
⌘ Campaigns to raise awareness of recommended levels and the harms associated with alcohol misuse.
⌘ Targeting high-risk or vulnerable groups (professional women, young people, young black men, binge drinkers).
⌘ Media campaigns ('Don't drink and drive', 'Don't drink whilst operating machinery' etc).
⌘ Shatterproof glasses in pubs.
⌘ Training of professionals to identify and respond to alcohol-related health and social problems.
⌘ Training of those who serve in pubs or entertainment venues to identify and refuse drunken customers.
⌘ Placing a ban on street drinking.

Tips on cutting down

- ⌘ Write down each day how much you drink (in units) — seeing it in black and white helps.
- ⌘ If there is a situation in which you always have a drink — for example, after work — try to cut it out.
- ⌘ When out for the evening, don't drink more than one drink an hour. Set yourself a maximum — say, two or three drinks — and stick to it.
- ⌘ Sip any alcoholic drink slowly; savour the aroma and flavour; make it last longer.
- ⌘ Always make your first drink a thirst-quenching soft one.
- ⌘ Try one of the many varieties of refreshing low-alcohol or, better still, non-alcoholic drinks.
- ⌘ Dilute alcoholic drinks with mixers: have a spritzer rather than wine on its own; avoid neat spirits; have a shandy rather than a beer.
- ⌘ Don't get into round-buying.
- ⌘ Say 'No' every so often.

Sources: Alcohol Concern: www.alcoholconcern.org.uk/servlets/doc/61; www.kca.org.uk/Leaflets/LFT_Cutting%20down.htm; www.nhsdirect.wales.nhs.uk/nhsdirect.asp?id=290 (all last accessed January 2005)

Useful websites (all last accessed January 2005)

Alcohol Concern — information on all aspects of alcohol and drinking www.alcoholconcern.org.uk

Alcoholics Anonymous — local self-help groups for drinkers and their families www.alcoholics-anonymous.org.uk

LifeBytes — the alcohol section of the Wired for Health site LifeBytes for Key Stage 3 pupils contains information on alcohol and health and legal issues. There is an interactive quiz (Flash plug-in required) and ideas for further activities: www.lifebytes.gov.uk/alcohol/alc_menu.html

Portman Group — a pan-industry organisation whose purpose is to help prevent misuse of alcohol and promote sensible drinking: www.portman-group.org.uk/

References

Alcohol Concern (2003) Alcohol and Mortality. http://www.alcoholconcern.org.uk/files/20030807_172030_mortality.pdf (last accessed January 2005)

Ambrogne JA (2002) Reduced-risk drinking as a treatment goal: what clinicians need to know. *J Subst Abuse Treat* **22**: 45–53

Ashworth M, Gerada C (1997) ABC of mental health: addiction and dependence-II: alcohol. *BMJ* **315**: 358–60

Beinhart S, Anderson B, Lee S, Utting D (2002) *Youth at risk? A national survey of risk factors, protective factors and problem behaviour among young people in England, Scotland and Wales.* London: Communities That Care

Cabinet Office (2003) Alcohol Misuse: How much does it cost? London: Cabinet Office Strategy Unit. http://www.number10.gov.uk/files/pdf/econ.pdf (last accessed January 2005)

Coleman JC, Hendry LB (1999) *Adolescent Health.* 3rd ed. London: Routledge

DoH (1999) *Reducing Health Inequalities: an Action Report.* London: DoH

DoH (2001a) *Smoking, Drinking and Drug Use Among Young People in England in 2000.* London: HMSO

DoH (2001b) *Statistics on Alcohol: England 1978 Onwards. Statistical Bulletin 2001/3.* London: DoH

DoH (2001c) *Annual Report of the Chief Medical Officer.* London: DoH

DoH (2003) Statistics on Alcohol in England 2003. London: DoH. http://www.publications.doh.gov.uk/public/sb0320.pdf (last accessed January 2005)

Engineer R, Phillips A, Thompson J, Nicolls J (2003) Drunk and Disorderly: a Qualitative Study of Binge Drinking Among 18 to 24 Year Olds. Home Office Research: Development and Statistics Directorate. http://www.homeoffice.gov.uk/rds/pdfs2/hors262.pdf (last accessed January 2005)

Guest JF, Varney S (2001) *Alcohol Misuse in Scotland: Trends and Costs.* Edinburgh: Scottish Executive Health Department

Health Development Agency (2004) Binge Drinking in the UK and on the Continent. http://www.hda.nhs.uk/downloads/pdfs/choosing_health/CHB8-binge-drinking.pdf (last accessed January 2005)

Institute of Alcohol Studies (2004a) Alcohol Consumption and Harm in the UK and EU. http://www.ias.org.uk/factsheets/harm-ukeu.pdf (last accessed January 2005)

Institute of Alcohol Studies (2004b) Binge Drinking: Nature, Prevalence and Causes. http://www.ias.org.uk/factsheets/binge-drinking.pdf (last accessed January 2005)

Institute of Alcohol Studies (2005) Young People and Alcohol. http://www.ias.org.uk/factsheets/young-people.pdf (last accessed January 2005)

Lader D, Meltzer H (2001) *Drinking: Adults' Behaviour and Knowledge in 2000.* London: Office for National Statistics Social Survey

Leech P (undated) *Current Developments in Primary Care.* London: DoH

Lintonen TP, Konu AI, Rimpela M (2001) Identifying potential heavy drinkers in early adolescence. *Health Educ* **101**(4): 159–68

Makela K, Mustonen H (2000) Relationships of drinking behaviour, gender and age with reported negative and positive experiences related to drinking. *Addiction* **95**(5): 727–36

Norman P, Bennett P, Lewis H (1998) Understanding binge drinking among young people: an application of the theory of planned behaviour. *Health Educ Res* **13**(2): 163–9

Office for National Statistics (2003) *Health Statistics Quarterly*. London: HMSO

Purser B, Orford J, Johnson M (2001) *Drinking in Second and Subsequent Black and Asian Communities in the English Midlands*. London: Alcohol Concern

Royal College of Physicians (2002) *Alcohol — Can the NHS Afford it? A Report of a Working Party of the Royal College of Physicians*. London: RCP

Waller S, Naidoo B, Thom B (2002) Prevention and reduction of alcohol misuse: evidence briefing. London: NHS Health Development Agency

White A (2001a) *Report on the Scoping Study on Men's Health*. London: DoH

Wise P, Pietroni R, Wilkes S (1995) Alcoholism. www.surgerydoor.co.uk (accessed January 2005)

WHO (2002) The European Health Report. Copenhagen: WHO Europe

World Cancer Research Fund (undated) Alcoholic Drinks Factsheet. http://www.wcrf-uk.org/publications/leafletdetail.lasso?WCRFS=52299DE2030112030EJtm3A8D D1B&SN=7 (last accessed January 2005)

Chapter 5

Maintaining a healthy weight

Obesity is now reported as the second leading cause of preventable death after smoking.

ICN (www.icn.ch/FactSheets/matters_obesity.pdf accessed January 2005)

Globally, there are more than one billion overweight adults, at least 300 million of them obese. Obesity and overweight pose a major risk for chronic diseases, including type 2 diabetes, cardiovascular disease, hypertension and stroke, and certain forms of cancer. The key causes are increased consumption of energy-dense foods high in saturated fats and sugars and reduced physical activity.

World Health Organisation (WHO) (2003)

Obesity is associated with a reduction in life expectancy of approximately nine years, mostly due to an increased risk of cardiovascular disease and certain cancers. It also increased the burden of ill-health, in particular type 2 diabetes. Prevention of obesity is the key to reducing the long term burden of obesity-related disease.

British Heart Foundation (BHF) (2004)

Definition and prevalence of obesity

Obesity is a chronically relapsing and potentially life-threatening medical condition and a recognised contributor to a wide range of other serious health problems (www.nationalobesityforum.org.uk/all_party_parlim.htm accessed January 2005). Obesity occurs when a person's intake of energy repeatedly exceeds the amount of energy they expend. The rates of obesity in the UK have trebled in the last twenty years. In 2002, 45% of men and 33% of women in England were overweight and a further 21% of men and 22% of women were clinically obese (BHF, 2004; APHO 2005). This means that in 2002, there were almost twenty-four million overweight or obese adults (NICE, 2004). The highest rates of obesity in young men in England are in the north east and Yorkshire and Humber regions, where 40% are either obese or overweight (APHO, 2005). In Northern Ireland, 63% of men are either overweight or obese compared with 50% of women (McWhirter, 2002). It is predicted that by 2010, one in four adults in the UK will be obese, costing the economy about £3.6 billion (Parliamentary Office of Science and Technology [POST], 2003). The prevalence of obesity in the UK reflects a major health problem that affects all socio-economic classes (Adolfsson *et al*, 2005). In terms of ethnicity, Indian men living in the UK are more likely to be obese than other men living in the UK (APHO 2005).

The prevalence of obesity in schoolchildren is also increasing, which does not bode well for their future health (National Audit Office, 2001). Children who are Asian are four times more likely to be obese than their white peers (APHO, 2005). In Wales, obesity levels in fifteen year-olds are higher than those in Scotland and England (Parry-Langdon and Roberts, 2004). The 2001 estimates in England suggest about 8.5% of six year-olds and 15% of fifteen year-olds are obese, and there is a similar prevalence in Scotland (POST, 2003). 'However, the greatest increases in the levels of overweight and obesity are being seen in children aged zero to four years. In the 1998 Avon Longitudinal Study of Parents and Children (ALSPAC), 18.7% of five year-olds surveyed were overweight; 7.2% were obese' (POST, 2003: 3).

The UK has the unenviable accolade of having one of the developed world's fastest-growing rate of obesity, with only Kuwait and Samoa topping it (BHF, 2004). The causes for the increasing levels of obesity are:

⌘   Sedentary lifestyles with concomitant lack of exercise.
⌘   Devices that save us time, effort and labour.
⌘   High intake of energy-dense micronutrient-poor foods (fast foods).
⌘   High intake of sugary, fizzy, soft drinks and juices.
⌘   Large portion sizes.
⌘   Decline in children playing sport at school (46% of children spent two hours or more a week in 1994; 1999 figures are 33%).
⌘   Just over 50% of children walk to school (62% in 1999).
⌘   Children between the ages of four and fifteen spend on average more than 2.5 hours a day watching television.
⌘   In 2002, about 50% of children have internet access at home and on average log on ten times a month.

Sources: All-Party Parliamentary Group on Obesity (2003a); POST (2003)

There is a noticeable socioeconomic dimension to being overweight and obese. Kennedy (2001) reports that research consistently shows that low-income households find it difficult to adopt healthy eating guidelines. This, Kennedy explains, is not due to a lack of knowledge of what constitutes a healthy diet, but rather economic and circumstantial barriers such as lack of income, lack of access to shops and/or a lack of access to storage or cooking facilities.

Inchley *et al* (2001) assert that children from more affluent families eat more fruit and vegetables than their less affluent counterparts, who consume more crisps, sweets, chocolate and fizzy drinks. The researchers also note that the greatest difference between these two groups is best seen in the consumption of chips: 58% of children from less affluent families ate chips daily compared with their more affluent counterparts, of whom 29% ate chips daily.

Parmenter *et al* (2000) carried out a survey of 1040 individuals to examine the nutrition knowledge and demographic variations in knowledge in a wide cross-section of adults in England. The first section of the questionnaire related to dietary recommendations. Results indicated that more than 90% were aware of recommendations to reduce the intake of fat, sugar and salt, and to increase the intake of fruit, vegetables and fibre. However, a number were unaware of other recommendations: to reduce the intake of saturated fat (25%); to reduce the intake of meat (51%); and to eat more starchy carbohydrates (90%). Furthermore, 70% could not state the recommended daily intake of fruit and vegetables and just over 50% thought that three (rather than five) portions a day was adequate.

Knowledge related to food groups was the second section of the questionnaire. Findings revealed that their knowledge about fibre was satisfactory but about 50% were unaware that cheese was high in salt, and the majority had poor knowledge about monounsaturated fat, with less than 2% knowing that olive oil contains mostly this type of fat.

The section on diet and disease relationships revealed that almost 15% were unaware of the link between a high fat intake and disease, but those that were aware of the link knew it could cause heart disease. Parmenter *et al* (2000) report that 41% of the survey sample were unaware of the consequences of developing health problems and a low intake of fruit and vegetables. Only 42% knew that eating more fruit and vegetables can help to reduce the risk of cancer and 47% knew it could also reduce the risk of coronary heart disease. The link between a high salt intake and cardiovascular problems was identified by 84%. Most of the sample thought that sugar could cause diabetes and obesity, but only about 25% mentioned tooth decay. The poorest item in this section was that only 22% of respondents had ever heard of antioxidants. Women had a slightly greater level of knowledge than men did. And it was noted that those in the youngest age group scored lower than those in middle years, with those aged over sixty-five obtaining the lowest scores. Finally, individuals who were married or living together achieved slightly higher scores than those who were single, separated, divorced or widowed (Parmenter *et al*, 2000).

Rather worryingly, since Parmenter *et al*'s (2000) study, Cancer Research UK (2005) reported from their survey of over 4000 people that 66% of those questioned were unaware that being obese or overweight increased their risk of cancer, and 67% were unaware that having a diet low in fruit and vegetables also increased their chance of developing cancer.

Box 5.1: Key facts about overweight and obesity

⌘ Children who are obese are at increased risk of developing physical health problems such as those associated with the cardiovascular system, obstructive sleep apnoea, asthma and orthopaedic problems with their feet and knees. Additionally, obese children are at risk of developing psychological problems (often associated with the stigma of being fat) such as low self-esteem, lack of confidence and depression.

⌘ A child who develops type I diabetes before the age of seven reduces their life expectancy by an average of 18%.

⌘ It is thought that increasing levels of obesity in children contribute to the increasing numbers of children and young people developing type I diabetes (rates have doubled in the last twenty years) and type II diabetes.

⌘ A fifty-year old man, already overweight at the age of eighteen, hastwice the risk of mortality compared with someone of healthy weight. forty year-old obese non-smoker reduces their life expectancy by 6.5 years; an obese individual who also smokes reduces their life expectancy by just over thirteen years.

⌘ The cost to the NHS of treating obesity-related health problems exceeds £2 billion.

⌘ Obesity and overweight have been associated with increased risk of developing certain types of cancer — of the colon, kidney, oesophagus, prostate and rectum.

⌘ It is estimated that roughly 33% of cancers could be avoided by adopting healthy eating and exercising patterns in order to maintain a healthy body weight throughout life.

Sources: POST (2003) www.nationalobesityforum.org.uk/all_party_parlim.htm
(accessed January 2005); WHO (2003a, b)

Measurement of obesity

The body mass index (BMI) is the international standard for assessing weight. It is based on the 1869 observations of a Belgian astronomer who postulated that people of a normal build had a weight that was proportional to the square of their height (www.malehealth.co.uk/userpage1.cfm?item_id=137 accessed February 2005). An online calculator to work out an individual's BMI can be found at www.nhlbisupport.com/bmi (accessed February 2005). The BMI is calculated in three steps:

1. Work out your height in metres and square it (ie. multiply the figure by itself).
2. Measure your weight in kilogrammes.
3. Divide your weight by the height squared.

The malehealth website provides the following example: a person is 5 ft 10 inch (1.78 m) and weighs 13 stone (82 kg). So 1.78 x 1.78 = 3.17. The BMI is thus 82 / 3.17 = 26. So the person's BMI is 26 — but what does that mean? WHO (2003a,b) provides the following information:

Table 5.1: BMI and risk of disease		
BMI	**Classification**	**Risk of disease associated with excess weight**
Less than 18.5	Underweight	Low (but increased risk of other clinical problems)
18.5–24.9	Desirable or normal range	Average
25–29.9	Overweight	Increased
30–34.9	Obese (Class I)	Moderate
35–39.9	Obese (Class II)	Severe
Over 40	Morbidly or severely obese (Class III)	Very severe

Men are more likely than women to be overweight (*Table 5.2*):

Table 5.2: BMI in England, 2001				
	Underweight	**Desirable weight**	**Overweight**	**Obese**
Males (16+)	4%	28%	47%	21%
Females (16+)	6%	38%	33%	23%

Source: Office for National Statistics (2004) cited at:
http://www.statistics.gov.uk/cci/nugget.asp?id=439
(last accessed February 2005)

The distribution of the extra fat is significant in terms of predicting risk to the individual. The health risks are compounded if the excess fat is distributed around the waist (central obesity). In general, men are at risk of obesity-related diseases when the waist circumference reaches 94 cm (37 inches) and becomes substantially increased if the waist size is 102 cm (40 inches) (National Audit Office, 2001; Melin and Rossner, 2003). The National Audit Office (2001) report states that in 1998, 19% of adults in England had a BMI over thirty. Forty-six percent of men were classed as overweight and 17% of men were classed as obese. South Asian men have higher levels of central obesity than men in the general population. Chinese and Black Caribbean men have significantly lower rates than those in the general population (DoH, 1999).

Diseases attributed to obesity

A man with a BMI of 22–23 is about half as likely to suffer from CHD than a man with a BMI > 30 and he is eight times less likely to develop diabetes. This problem will worsen as men become increasingly sedentary and eat a high-fat diet.

Baker (2001: 4)

Obesity is a significant avoidable risk factor for a range of serious and chronic diseases:

- cardiovascular disease
- hypertension and stroke (being 3.5 stone overweight increases the risk of developing hypertension by 700%)
- high blood levels of cholesterol
- gastro-intestinal and liver disease
- type II diabetes (non-insulin-dependent; being 3.5 stone overweight increases the risk of developing diabetes by 3000%)
- various forms of cancer
- musculoskeletal problems
- varicose veins
- gall-bladder disease
- sleep apnoea
- depression and accidents

Source: (ICN, 2002: http://www.man-health-magazine-online. com/health-man.html accessed February 2005)

Of all the serious diseases, type II diabetes has the strongest association with obesity. The clearest association of obesity with cancer is that of colon cancer and there is evidence that it increases the risk of prostate and rectal cancer in men (National Audit Office, 2001; APHO, 2005). The European Health Report (WHO, 2002b) states that obese men are more likely than non-obese men to die from cancer of the colon, rectum and prostate.

Diets high in salt are likely to increase the risk of developing gastric cancer; those high in red meat probably increase the risk of colorectal and prostate cancer; and diets high in fat may increase the risk of cancer developing in the lung, colon, rectum and prostate. Increased weight will increase the stress on weight-bearing joints, particularly those in the lower extremities, which leads to osteoarthritis. A BMI of 30 or more markedly increases the risk for osteoarthritis of the knees.

According to Sky News Online (2003), someone who is overweight at forty years of age is likely to die at least three years earlier than their counterpart who is not overweight, which makes this risk factor as bad as smoking in terms of life expectancy. The same source reports that obese men on average live 5.8 years less and obese women live 7.1 years less. It has also been reported that an obese person who is otherwise physically fit has a lower mortality risk than an obese person who has a low level of cardio-respiratory fitness (National Audit Office, 2001).

The National Audit Office report *Tackling Obesity in England* (2001: 14) states that obesity not only causes the conditions cited above, but also significant psychological and social burdens: 'social stigma, low self-esteem, reduced mobility and a generally poorer quality of life are common experiences for many obese people.'

Table 5.3: Estimated increased risk for the obese of developing associated diseases (taken from international studies)

Disease	Relative risk: women	Relative risk: men
Type II diabetes	12.7	5.2
Hypertension	4.2	2.6
Myocardial infarction (heart attack)	3.2	1.5
Cancer of the colon	2.7	3.0
Angina	1.8	1.8
Gall bladder disease	1.8	1.8
Ovarian cancer	1.7	—
Osteoarthritis	1.4	1.9
Stroke	1.3	1.3

Source: National Audit Office (2001)

Type II diabetes

An estimated 135 million people worldwide had diagnosed diabetes in 1995, and this number is expected to rise to at least 300 million by 2025.

Narayan *et al* (2001: 63)

The increase in type II diabetes mirrors the increase in the proportion of people, including children and young people, who are either overweight or obese.

DoH (2001: 16)

In England, there are 1.3 million people diagnosed with diabetes (DoH, 2001). In Scotland, there are about 150,000 people who have diabetes and there are thousands more who are undiagnosed. It is anticipated that the number for Scotland may double in the next ten to fifteen years (NHS Scotland, 2005).

Diabetes mellitus is a chronic, progressive, degenerative disease. There are two types of diabetes: type I and type II. Type I is also known as insulin-dependent diabetes. Individuals with type I diabetes are unable to make insulin for themselves. The usual onset for type I diabetes is in childhood and individuals with this condition must inject insulin daily. Type II diabetes is also known as non-insulin-dependent diabetes. It develops when the body still produces some insulin, but either not enough or the insulin produced doesn't work properly.

Diabetes has been defined as:

A condition where there is a shortage of, or an inability to respond to, insulin. Insulin is a hormone produced by the pancreas, which is needed to transport glucose (sugar) obtained from food, from the bloodstream into the body's cells where it is converted into energy. This results in a build up of glucose in the blood (hyperglycaemia).

(NHS Scotland, 2004: 13)

The main symptoms of untreated diabetes are: an increased thirst, which causes individuals to drink more fluid than they would otherwise, which in turn causes frequent trips to the toilet, especially at night; genital itching; a feeling of extreme tiredness; blurred vision; and weight loss. The clinical signs of diabetes are glycosuria (glucose in the urine) and a fasting blood glucose greater than 7 mmol/L (Burden, 2003).

Onset and prevalence of type II diabetes

*Excess weight gain, overweight and obesity and physical inactivity
account for the escalating rates of type II diabetes, worldwide.
Diabetes leads to increased risk of heart disease, kidney disease,
stroke and infections. Increased physical activity and maintaining a
healthy weight play critical roles in the prevention and treatment of
diabetes.*

WHO (2003)

*Type II diabetes usually has no symptoms, but in the long term it
can lead to excessive thirst, frequent trips to the toilet to pass urine,
and weight loss. Type II diabetes can usually be controlled with diet,
exercise or medicines, but if poorly controlled, it increases the risk of
heart disease and strokes, nerve damage and blindness.*

BUPA (2003)

The usual onset for type II diabetes is after the age of forty. The onset is often insidious and it is thought that, on average, people can have type II diabetes for six to seven years before it is diagnosed (Burden, 2003). Those at risk of developing type II diabetes are those who are overweight, physically inactive or have a family history of the disease. People of South Asian descent are six times more likely than white people to develop type II diabetes; those of African or African-Caribbean descent are three times more likely (DoH, 2001).

In England, the frequency of type II diabetes is higher in men than in women (DoH, 2001). 'Most people with diabetes (about 85%) have type II, the number of people increasing with age and ethnicity. Ten percent of the UK white population over the age of sixty-five years have type II diabetes. The numbers are even higher in the Indo-Asian population — at least 25% of those over the age of sixty-five have type II diabetes' (Burden, 2003: 30). Type II diabetes is more prevalent among the less affluent population. The DoH (2001) states that those in the most deprived fifth of the population are 1.5 times more likely to develop type II diabetes. Morbidity arising from type II diabetes is 3.5 times higher in the poorest people in our society compared with the most affluent (DoH, 2001).

Type II diabetes and links to obesity

The cause of type II diabetes has long been linked to behavioural and environmental factors such as excess weight, physical inactivity and dietary habits (Narayan *et al*, 2001). In 2002, Dyer reported that the first diagnosed cases of type II diabetes mellitus in clinically obese children had been made in three girls aged from thirteen to fifteen and a boy aged fifteen. Type II diabetes is positively associated with the level and duration of obesity and body-fat distribution (NELH, 2001). Excessive body weight reduces the body's ability to respond to insulin, which explains why excess weight and obesity are risk factors for the development of type II diabetes (DoH, 2001).

Complications of type II diabetes

The consequence of type II diabetes is that it reduces quality of life in the form of acute metabolic complications; hyperlipidaemia; hypertension; peripheral vascular disease; blindness; and neuropathy (Koch *et al*, 2000). Diabetes is the leading cause of blindness in people of working age; the largest single cause of end-stage renal failure; and the biggest cause of lower-limb amputation. Cataracts tend to develop ten years earlier in diabetics than they do in non-diabetics. Cataracts are also twice as common in diabetics (DoH, 2001).

The life expectancy of individuals with type II diabetes is reduced on average by ten years — their mortality rate from coronary heart disease is about five times higher and the risk of suffering a stroke is three times higher than non-diabetics (DoH, 2001). Some ethnic groups have a greater risk of developing type II diabetes. These groups have a greater risk of death from complications of the disease — the risk is between three and six times higher, probably because they are particularly susceptible to the cardiovascular and renal complications (DoH, 2001).

Reducing the risk of developing type II diabetes

The onset of type II diabetes can be delayed, or even prevented, by eating a healthy diet, losing weight and increasing the level of physical activity (DoH, 2001). Increasing physical activity in type II diabetics has the effect of normalising the effect of body weight, blood pressure and the lipoprotein profile (Batty *et al*, 2002).

Prevention of obesity

Tell me what you eat, and I will tell you what you are.
Anthelme Brillat-Savarin (1755–1826)

> *Obesity reduces life expectancy by an average of nine years.*
>
> (APHO, 2005)

> *Obesity and overweight may account for 14% of male cancer deaths and 20% of female cancer deaths.*
>
> (APHO, 2005)

For normal adults to maintain a healthy body weight, they need to limit their calorie intake to ten calories per pound (lb) of their weight. Thus, a person weighing 150 lbs needs about 1500 calories per day to avoid gaining weight.

Young adults can generally eat more and not gain weight, but metabolism tends to slow down in the mid-thirties. That, coupled with a trend that those in their mid-thirties tend to be less active than they were in their younger years, leads to many adults gaining weight.

Adopting a lifestyle that includes a healthy diet and exercise is the key to preventing the development of obesity. However, once someone is overweight or obese, losing weight can be difficult — but desirable, given the known health gains. To lose one pound of body fat, one needs an energy deficit of 3,500 calories.

Crawford (2002: 728) writes:

> *To prevent obesity, health authorities have proposed a series of population-based strategies that place an emphasis on changing the environment. These include strategies such as modifying the design of buildings to encourage the use of stairs; examining urban design to make neighbourhoods more walkable; promoting active transport by providing a safer and more integrated network of footpaths and bicycle lanes; improving food labelling to help consumers make informed choices; and increasing the range of healthy foods in schools and work cafeterias.*

Drummond (2002) advocates that advice given to obese individuals must be perceived as being achievable and therefore small changes to their diet is the most acceptable approach. She provides the following achievable changes:

- Choose low-fat or reduced-fat dairy products — for example, change from full-fat to semi-skimmed milk, or from semi-skimmed to skimmed milk.
- Change from frying foods to grilling, baking, boiling or steaming.
- Choose lean meats and trim all visible fat off meat before cooking.
- Avoid all spreadable fats — instead, use a thin layer of jam on toast, scones and so on, and avoid completely on sandwiches.

⌘ Limit intakes of food high in hidden fats — for example, meat pies. Instead, choose meat stews with extra vegetables.

⌘ Choose tomato-based sauces for pasta/rice instead of cream or cheese sauces.

⌘ Choose low-fat savoury snacks such as pretzels, Twiglets and rice crackers, instead of nuts and crisps.

Why reduce fat?

According to the National Audit Office (2001: 18), 'exposure to high-fat foods is thought to be largely responsible for the "over-eating effect" also known as "passive over-consumption" where the appetite fails to regulate adequately the amount of energy consumed.' Fats add taste and texture to food, making it particularly palatable and addictive. Fats seem to promote a reduced sense of satiety or fullness compared with protein-rich or carbohydrate-rich foods. The result is that more calories are eaten to achieve the same fullness feeling that comes from proteins and carbohydrates (Satia-Abouta *et al*, 2002). Calorie for calorie, fat is less filling than carbohydrate (Drummond, 2002).

There are four different types of fat: polyunsaturated, monounsaturated, saturated and trans-fats. They can be differentiated by their chemical structure (WHO, 2003a). Saturated fats such as lard have a hard or solid consistency, whilst polyunsaturated fats such as sunflower oil are liquids. All foods and oils contain a mixture of fats and not just one type. Details about the four different types of fat can be seen at www.wcrf-uk.org/publications/informeddetail.lasso; http://www.malehealth.co.uk/userpage1.cfm?item_id=148 (both accessed January 2005).

Polyunsaturated fats

⌘ Some essential polyunsaturated fats must be consumed in food because the body cannot make them — examples are linoleic acid (omega 6 family) and alpha-linolenic acid (omega 3 family).

⌘ Polyunsaturated fats are required for growth, the structure of cell membranes and the production of chemical messengers which help regulate functions such as blood clotting, blood pressure and immunity.

⌘ In moderation, omega 6 fats help lower blood cholesterol levels.

⌘ Good sources of omega 6 fats include sunflower, corn and safflower oils and margarines; grapeseed oil; and sunflower and sesame seeds.

⌘ Good sources of omega 3 fats include oily fish (mackerel, salmon, kippers, trout, sardines); rapeseed oil; soya oil and spread; walnut

oils; pumpkin seeds; linseeds; wholegrains; walnuts; and sweet potatoes.
- ⌘ Some research shows that the balance between omega 3 and some omega 6 acids may help to protect against cancer.
- ⌘ The omega 3 and omega 6 groups are already known to be involved in protecting against or easing arthritis and cardiovascular disease.

Monosaturated fats

- ⌘ In moderation, monosaturated fats help lower blood cholesterol levels, especially when they are eaten in place of saturated fats.
- ⌘ Good sources include peanut oil; olive oil and olive oil-based spreads; rapeseed oil; avocados; and most nuts.
- ⌘ The majority of vegetable oils that don't specify a fat source are usually rapeseed oils, and therefore a cheap source of monosaturates.

Saturated fats

- ⌘ Eating too many saturates causes the liver to make more bad low-density lipoprotein (LDL) cholesterol; this raises cholesterol levels, which are linked to the development of heart disease.
- ⌘ Saturated fats incorporated into the blood cells can make them more 'sticky', thereby increases the risk of developing blood clots (thrombosis).
- ⌘ Saturated fats increase the risk of developing atherosclerosis, whereby the insides of the blood vessels 'fur' up. This furring up narrows the lumen of the blood vessel, which in turn reduces the blood flow supplied by the blood vessels. In the coronary blood vessels, this can lead to the symptoms of angina and in the peripheral blood vessels it leads to peripheral vascular disease and the symptoms of intermittent claudication. As the blood vessels fur up, there is increased turbulence in the blood flow, which can lead to an increased risk of clot formation and damage to the integrity of the wall of the blood vessel, which can result in the formation of an aneurysm.
- ⌘ Saturated fats are mostly found in animal foods such as fatty meat, cheese, butter and cream. They are also found in palm and coconut oils; pies; biscuits; and cakes. Fatty processed and fast foods are additional sources.

Trans-fats

⌘ Trans-fats are formed when unsaturated fats are bombarded with hydrogen to make them more saturated (a process called hydrogenation) so that they will be firmer and last longer. As well as creating more saturated fats, hydrogenation forms trans-fats.

⌘ Like saturated fats, too many trans-fats can raise blood cholesterol levels.

⌘ The main sources of trans-fats are margarines; spreads; processed foods, such as pies and pastries; and fast foods. They are also found in any food ingredients labelled 'hydrogenated vegetable oils/fats'.

⌘ Very small amounts occur naturally in butter, full-fat milk and meat.

Changing dietary habits and behaviour

Having the knowledge about what makes up a healthy diet is one thing — but to be effective, it has to be accompanied by a change in dietary habits and behaviours. The latter can be very difficult. There is increasing evidence that dietary habits established in childhood are very difficult to change in adulthood (Inchley *et al*, 2001). This is reinforced by Caroli and Lagravinese (2002) and APHO (2005) who state that child and adolescent obesity is associated with being overweight and obese in adulthood. Inchley *et al* (2001) and Caroli and Lagravinese (2002) call for continued health promotion efforts in improving the diet of children, thereby preventing adult obesity and morbidity. Inchley *et al* (2001) note that almost 33% of Scottish children still don't eat fruit daily and about 50% don't eat vegetables daily. The average fruit and vegetable consumption in England is about three portions a day, but this figure is lower in children and those on low incomes (APHO, 2005). Caroli and Lagravinese (2002: 223) report that 'infants who were breastfed for longer periods showed a significant lower risk of being overweight during childhood and adolescence than infants who were fed mostly with formula or were breastfed for less than three months.' They conclude that five modifying factors are key to the prevention of obesity:

1. Increase breastfeeding in terms of percentage and duration.
2. Modify wrong weaning patterns by decreasing protein intake and by increasing fat intake until two years of age.
3. Modify the eating habits of toddler and school-age children by decreasing fat intake and increasing carbohydrates and fibre intake.

4. Help parents and/or guardians to understand the real needs of their children without using foods as a form of gratification, reward and/or consolation for every negative feeling and situation.
5. Ask governments, consumer unions, food industries and mass media to reduce and regulate non-nutritional food advertising during children's television time.

Kennedy (2001) advocates changes in the physical and social environment to facilitate lifestyle changes. There are a number of barriers associated with eating a more healthy diet. A population survey found lack of will power was identified by 35%; followed by health foods being too expensive (25%); not liking the taste of healthy foods (15%); and not knowing what changes to make (15%). Men most commonly cited the latter two barriers. Related to will power is self-efficacy, which relates to the person's perceptions of whether they will achieve their goal or not. If they believe that attaining the goal will be relatively easy and that they will have a degree of control over the change in their behaviour, they are more likely to succeed. For this reason, Povey *et al* (2000) suggest that strategies aiming to promote health-related changes in diet would benefit by targeting people's attitudes and their self-efficacy over the change.

Table 5.4: Identification of barriers to healthy eating and examples of interventions to address them	
Barrier	**Intervention**
Belief that the family is already eating enough fruit and vegetables	Information about five portions a day and portion sizes
Dislike of vegetables and lack of confidence in cooking and preparing them; fear of waste and rejection by the family	Set up cooking-skills clubs and tasting sessions, or develop cooking sessions as part of the activities of existing groups (eg. women's groups, youth groups)
Difficulty in finding affordable, good-quality fruit and vegetables locally	Set up community-owned retailing and food co-operatives to introduce affordable supplies

Source: *Coronary Heart Disease: Guidelines for Implementing the Preventative Aspects of the National Service Framework* (2000)

Parmenter (2002) offers some additional suggestions to overcome barriers: fruit and vegetables are inexpensive if bought in season; eat fruit as snacks, on top of cereal; and make healthy eating fun for children by using, for example, vegetables with dips.

It is generally accepted that a healthy diet should be made up of less than 30% fat. There are several sources of information related to how to eat less fat (www.jr2.ox.ac.uk/bandolier/booth/hliving/loswt.html, accessed February 2005; Maintaining a Healthy Body Weight: http://www.wcrf-uk.org/publications/leafletdetail.lasso?WCRFS=52299DE2030112030EJtm3A8DD1B&SN=24, accessed February 2005) and the information is combined in the following information:

⌘ Choose a low or reduced fat spread and use it sparingly, if at all.
⌘ Try not to use any spread when it may not be necessary.
⌘ Eat less meat and meat products. Choose the leanest meat available and trim off all visible fat before cooking.
⌘ Opt for fish or poultry as a healthy alternative to red meat and remember to remove skin from poultry: 3 oz of roast chicken with skin contains 12 g of fat; without skin, the fat content falls to 5 g.
⌘ Opt for low-fat dairy products such as skimmed or semi-skimmed milk (both have just as much calcium and protein as whole milk, but much less fat); reduced-fat cheeses; and low-fat yoghurts and fromage frais. Per pint, whole milk has 22 g of fat; semi-skimmed has 9 g; and skimmed milk has 0.6 g. One oz of double cream contains 14 g of fat; 1 oz low-fat plain yoghurt or low-fat fromage frais contains 0.3 g.
⌘ Try making salad dressings with natural yoghurt rather than mayonnaise or salad cream.
⌘ Choose raw vegetables such as carrot or celery sticks or fresh fruits instead of fatty snacks, sweets and cakes.
⌘ Bake, boil, steam, microwave, stir-fry or grill foods rather than frying or roasting them in fat. Three oz of fried cod in batter contains 9 g of fat; 3 oz of poached cod contains 1 g of fat.
⌘ Read nutrition labels in the shops and as a rough guide choose ready-meal and snack foods with less than 3 g of fat per 100 calories.

Weight reduction through drug therapy

Drugs such as Orlistat and Sibutramine are used in treating obesity in adults. The UK National Institute of Clinical Excellence (NICE) is currently reviewing its guidelines for these drugs and will cover adults and children aged over two years old. As well as including adults and children whose weight has already caused illness or those with or without risk factors for other medical conditions, the revised guideline will consider black and minority ethnic groups; lower socioeconomic groups; and vulnerable groups including older people and women of child-bearing age.

(NICE, 2004)

Impact of weight reduction on health

The HDA (2003) provides information on the improvements in health as a result of a modest weight reduction of 10kg:

- over 20% fall in total mortality
- over 30% fall in diabetes-related deaths
- over 40% fall in obesity-related cancer deaths
- fall of 10mmHg in systolic blood pressure and a fall of 20mmHg in diastolic blood pressure
- in newly diagnosed diabetics, a 50% fall in fasting blood glucose
- fall of 10% total cholesterol, 15% fall in low-density lipoprotein, and 30% fall in triglycerides
- improved lung function (reduction in central obesity)
- reduced back and joint pains

The World Cancer Research Research Fund UK state that if all of us ate five portions of fruit and vegetables daily, the overall cancer rates would be reduced by more than 20%. Combining dietary changes with not smoking has the potential to reduce cancer risk by 60–70% (Maintaining a Healthy Body Weight: http://www.wcrf-uk.org/publications/leafletdetail.lasso?WCRFS=5229 9DE2030112030EJtm3A8DD1B&SN=24, accessed February 2005).

To be successful in losing weight requires a holistic approach, incorporating behaviour modification, a healthy diet and physical activity. Success is dependent on a belief that the loss of weight is actually achievable, motivation, and an understanding of how to achieve that goal (Adolfsson *et al*, 2005), along with the realisation that just as it took time to put weight on, it takes time, patience and persistent to take it off.

Physical activity

Physical activity is a broad term to describe movement of the body that uses energy.

Scottish Executive (2002: 8)

The human species was designed for movement… our bodies have an inherent need to be exercised.

Sparling *et al* (2000: 367)

Over the past twenty to thirty years, there has been a decease in physical activity as part of the daily routines in England but a small increase in the proportion of people taking physical activity for leisure. Total miles travelled per year by foot fell by 26% and miles travelled by bicycle also fell by 26% (1975/6–1999/2001 National Travel Survey). This produced a difference of 66 miles walked per year between 1975–6 and 1999–2001. Twenty-five years ago, we walked nearly three marathons a year more than we do now. For a person weighing 65kg, this represents an annual reduction in energy expenditure equivalent to almost 1kg of fat.

(DoH, 2004a: 138)

The Exercise Alliance (2001) reports activity levels of the British adult population over two time frames (*Table 5.5*):

Table 5.5: Levels of physical activity of the British adult population in 1992 and 1998		
	Men	**Women**
1992	70% not active enough to gain health benefits	80% not active enough to gain health benefits
1998	37% meeting guidelines	25% meeting guidelines
	> 33% remain sedentary*	

*'Sedentary' means that the individual does less than one session of thirty minutes' moderate activity per week.

There is a variation in physical activity levels in different ethnic populations. Black-Caribbean men and white men are more than twice as likely to reach the recommended level of activity followed by Indian, Chinese, Pakistani and Bangladeshi men (POST, 2001).

In Scotland, 72% of women and 59% of men are not active enough; and 27% of boys and 40% of girls are not active enough. It is also noticeable that the proportion of sedentary adults in the lowest socioeconomic group is double that of the highest socioeconomic group (Scottish Executive, 2002). West *et al* (2002) report that one in three females in Glasgow said that they undertook no physical activity at all at age eighteen. This concurs with findings from Hunt *et al* (2001) who note that the levels of physical activity are generally low in the west of Scotland, which is also one of the areas of highest coronary morbidity and mortality.

Hussey *et al* (2001) state that, in Ireland in 1989, 33% of ten-to-thirteen year-olds exercised four or more times a week and 23% walked or cycled to school. In 1998, 58% of nine-to-seventeen year-olds exercised four or more times a week. It was noticeable that boys exercised more than girls, and that participation levels for both sexes decreased with age. The researchers highlighted the fact that 14% of boys and 24% of girls were not active enough to gain any health benefits.

Physical inactivity is estimated to cause, globally, about 10–16% of cases each of breast cancer, colon and rectal cancers and diabetes mellitus, and about 22% of ischaemic heart disease (WHO, 2002).

Risks of inactivity

⌘   A greater risk of heart attacks and strokes than active people.
⌘   Higher blood pressure (itself a major risk factor for heart disease).
⌘   A higher risk of developing some cancers.
⌘   More chance of developing diabetes.
⌘   A higher risk of osteoporosis, leading to fractures. Up to half of hip fractures could be avoided with regular physical activity.
⌘   Greater risk of being overweight or obese: this also increases the risk of other medical conditions.
⌘   More injuries and accidents than physically active people.
⌘   Inactive children are at risk of poorer self-esteem, greater anxiety and higher stress levels.
⌘   Inactive children are also more likely to smoke and use drugs than physically active children.
⌘   Inactive employees have more days off work than active employees.
⌘   In later life, inactive people lose the basic strength and flexibility for daily activities. As a result, many lose their independence and have poorer mental health.

Sources: Scottish Executive, 2003 (http://www.healthyliving.gov.uk/ physicalactivity/index.cfm?contentid=1346, accessed February 2005)

Benefits of physical activity

'The recommended amount of physical activity is to participate in at least thirty minutes of moderate-intensity physical activity on at least five days a week' (APHO, 2005). There is some evidence that some activity is better than no activity for gaining health benefits (Hall *et al*, 2002). According to UKWellness. com, the following benefits are accrued from physical activity:

•   heart attack is significantly reduced with 150Kcal of physical activity per day (100Kcal = roughly one mile of walking)
•   stroke is reduced by 20–40%

- diabetes type II is reduced by 30%
- hip fractures are reduced by 40%
- colon cancer is reduced by 10–46%
- stroke is reduced by 20–40%
- firmer muscle tone
- improved sleeping patterns
- increased metabolism
- increased ability to manage stress
- healthier heart and lungs
- stronger bones, which help prevent osteoporosis
- more energy
- prevention and/or elimination of lower back pain

UKWellness.com: http://www.ukwellness.com/medical-conditions/
risk/inactivity.html (accessed February 2005)

Promoting physical activity

*An active lifestyle is a key to better health. However, at present
only 31% of adults are sufficiently active to feel health benefits.
The challenge we now face is to encourage more people to become
active.*

(DoH 2004a)

The document *Choosing Health? Choosing Activity* (DoH, 2004a) specifies the
following activities over the lifespan of individuals:

- ⌘ Children and young people should achieve a total of at least sixty
  minutes of at least moderate-intensity physical activity each day.
- ⌘ Adults should achieve a total of at least thirty minutes a day of at
  least moderate-intensity physical activity on five or more days of the
  week.
- ⌘ For many people, forty-five to sixty minutes of moderate-intensity
  physical activity a day is necessary to prevent obesity.

The document stresses that the activities can be achieved in one session or by
breaking it up into ten-minute bouts of activity.

It is widely acknowledged that getting people to change their behaviour and
persuading them to become more physically active is a difficult task (Gillman
et al, 2001; Hunt *et al*, 2001; Van der Bij *et al*, 2002). In their research, which
focused on encouraging older people to become more active, Van der Bij *et
al* (2002) argue that any intervention should be tailored to the individual's
ideas and preferences. From their observational research, they also found

that individual factors such as motivation, social support, health, beliefs and education — as well as organisational factors such as resources, accessibility and type of physical activity — influence the success of an intervention.

The general consensus is that some activity is better than none at all (Hall *et al*, 2002) and that advocating moderate activity, as opposed to vigorous activity, is a more achievable goal (DoH, 2004b). Woolf-May *et al* (1999: 813) report the findings from their quantitative research study that 'fitness and health benefits may be gained from moderate-intensity exercise accumulated in fifteen-minute bouts during a day and could provide an effective exercise prescription for those who find it difficult to achieve the traditionally prescribed twenty-to-thirty minute prolonged bout of physical activity.'

Gillman *et al* (2001) found that increased amounts of physical activity were associated with a healthier diet and suggest that health promoters should target diet and activity together, as this strategy may attain enhanced outcomes. Hunt *et al* (2001) conclude that the types of physical activity that show long-term adherence are walking, swimming and social dancing. Regardless of the activity, Cale and Harris (2001) believe that the prime factor is enjoyment, as it has the strongest influence on activity levels.

Motivating individuals to increase their physical activity

> *Motivation is at the crux of health behaviour performance and thus, to a great extent, health. It is postulated that understanding motivation is the key to health promotion efforts of physical activity... Motivation is the intrinsic determination toward goal attainment.*

Plonczynski (2000: 695)

Woolf-May *et al* (1999) suggest that the establishment of exercise habits is an essential aspect of exercise participation and adherence. Generally speaking, the main thrust of the advice is to encourage intermittent daily activity of moderate intensity which is embedded as much as possible in normal daily life activities (WHO, 2002b), as it is through this that increased physical activity is more likely to become the norm for individuals (World Cancer Research Fund UK). Suggestions for incorporating physical activity into daily life are provided by www.loudtieday.org.uk (accessed January 2005). They suggest washing and waxing a car; washing windows or floors; hoovering; vigorous gardening or raking leaves; walking or jogging to work; cycling with the children; swimming or aqua aerobics; aerobics or keep fit classes; walking the dog.

A number of sources provide advice and tips on encouraging and sustaining motivation, which are summarised below:

Encouraging and sustaining motivation

- ⌘ Make friends with your body because if you see it as the enemy that needs to be punished, physical activity will always be a struggle.
- ⌘ Get fit for yourself.
- ⌘ Enjoy what you do; if you don't enjoy it, try something else.
- ⌘ If you get bored easily, change activities frequently to keep your mind alert and your body challenged.
- ⌘ Schedule at least three thirty-minute sessions as part of your weekly activities — don't let anything else take priority.
- ⌘ If cold weather is making you reluctant to leave your warm living-room, tell yourself you will only do ten minutes of running instead of twenty minutes, or fifteen minutes of weights instead of thirty. By the time you have done the small amount, you will probably have found the incentive to carry on.
- ⌘ Don't dwell on missed work-outs — put them behind you and focus on the future. You don't become unfit overnight.
- ⌘ Plan ahead by setting regular goals for yourself. Don't exercise aimlessly. Track your progress by keeping an exercise log and recording your weekly activity.
- ⌘ Motivate yourself by remembering how you feel after you have completed a work-out, and how good you feel knowing that you are taking good care of yourself.
- ⌘ Between 4pm and 6pm is probably the best time to go to the gym — studies have shown that evening exercisers are more likely to stick to their routines for longer.
- ⌘ Use exercise as a stress-management technique — walk to clear your head and help you make decisions.
- ⌘ Exercise with a friend or family member — it's sometimes easier when you have someone else encouraging you, and it is easier to keep the 'exercise habit' going because you have made a commitment.

Sources: www.malehealth.co.uk/feelbetter/exercise.htm;
WCRF UK http://wcrf-uk.org; www.loudtieday.org.uk
(all accessed January 2005)

Barriers to increasing physical activity

To improve people's physical activity, it is logical if we first look at the barriers that are put in the way. The barriers cited in the literature can be grouped under the headings of personal, social, cultural and environmental. *Table 5.6* shows the barriers to being more physically active by age (Scottish Executive, 2002).

It is estimated that only 34% of the Scottish population are aware of how much physical activity is required for good health (Scottish Executive, 2002).

Barriers	Age group in years					
	16–24	25–34	35–44	45–54	55–64	65–74
	%					
Preferring to do other things	36	24	16	16	18	9
Feeling too fat or overweight	11	18	10	14	15	17
Do not enjoy exercise	8	12	15	13	10	6
Being too old	3	1	3	9	8	21
Lack of time due to other commitments	58	71	71	53	37	21
Ill health, injury or disability	14	17	28	28	38	37
Lack of suitable local facilities	34	22	18	22	12	14
Lack of money	28	14	13	10	4	3
Lack of transport	11	14	4	5	2	6
Nobody to go with	32	15	21	14	6	7
Put off by traffic, road safety or environment	2	7	8	6	10	7
Put off by the weather	16	14	14	19	17	33
Don't have the skills or confidence to do it	9	6	8	8	5	9

Table 5.6: Barriers to being more physically active, by age

Source: Scottish Executive, 2002

In response to some of the perceived barriers to physical exercise, the WCRF UK make the following suggestions:

- ⌘ 'Too old — it's not age that determines physical fitness, it's desire. Whether you are twenty, fifty or ninety years old, you can improve your activity levels ands enjoy better mobility as well as independence. Remember, use it and improve it!
- ⌘ **Too busy** — try ten-minute 'bursts' of activity throughout the day to build up your total. It is estimated that three hours of life can be gained for every hour of exercise! And more importantly, quality of life is improved.
- ⌘ **Too tired** — next time you feel tired, go for a walk or a bike ride. Providing you aren't unwell, it will leave you feeling invigorated and, at the same time, improve your long-term resistance to colds and illness.
- ⌘ **Too unfit** — we all have to start somewhere — after all, it is difficult to be fit without exercising. No matter how unfit you think you are, you can always improve. You'll be congratulated, as well as respected, for even trying.'

Quick fitness tips for busy people

- ⌘ Use stationary activities as opportunities to work out your muscles. Flex your abdominals or clench your bottom whilst sitting at your desk or standing in a queue at the supermarket.
- ⌘ Do calf lifts while talking on the phone (probably better when you're on the home phone!)
- ⌘ Avoid taking the lift or escalator and always take the stairs — whether you are at work, on the Tube, in the shopping mall, etc.
- ⌘ Don't take the bus for short journeys — walk instead.
- ⌘ Offer to go to the post office or carry out office errands.
- ⌘ Do stretches in the shower — roll your neck, touch your toes, do shoulder shrugs.
- ⌘ Take advantage of your TV time. Do crunches or bicep curls with cans of baked beans while you watch *Coronation Street*! Get up from the sofa during commercial breaks and do jumping jacks.
- ⌘ Walk around the building during your lunch break. Wear a backpack to increase resistance.
- ⌘ Park farther away from building entrances.
- ⌘ If you don't have a dog, get one and walk it!
- ⌘ Plan holidays that include physical activity such as hiking, swimming or watersports.

Source: www.loudtieday.org.uk (accessed January 2003)

How individuals of different age-groups can achieve the recommended levels of activity

Table 5.7: How to achieve recommended levels of activity	
Age-group	**Activities**
Young child	Daily walk to and from school Daily school activity sessions (breaks and clubs) Three to four afternoon or evening play opportunities Weekend: longer walks, visits to park or swimming pool, bike rides
Teenager	Daily walk (or cycle) to and from school Three to four organised or informal midweek sports or activities Weekend: walks, biking, swimming, sports activities
Student	Daily walk (or cycle) to and from college Taking all small opportunities to be active: using stairs, doing manual tasks Two to three midweek student sports or exercise classes, visits to the gym or swimming pool Weekend: longer walks, biking, swimming, sports activities
Adult employed	Daily walk (or cycle) to and from work Taking all small opportunities to be active: using stairs, doing manual tasks Two to three midweek sport, gym or swimming sessions Weekend: longer walks, biking, swimming, sports activities, DIY, gardening
Adult houseworker	Daily walks, gardening or DIY Taking all small opportunities to be active: using stairs, doing manual tasks Occasional midweek sport, gym or swimming sessions Weekend: longer walks, biking, sports activities
Adult unemployed	Daily walks, gardening or DIY Taking all small opportunities to be active: using stairs, doing manual tasks Weekend: longer walks, biking, swimming, or sports activities Occasional sport, gym or swimming sessions
Retired person	Daily walking, cycling, DIY or gardening Taking all small opportunities to be active: using stairs, doing manual tasks Weekend: longer walks, biking or swimming

Source: *Physical Activity, Health Improvement and Prevention*
(DoH, 2004: 10)

Useful websites (all last accessed January 2005)

BBC Men's Health site — www.bbc.co.uk/health/mens/

British Dietetic Association — www.bda.uk.com

British Nutrition Foundation — www.nutrition.org.uk — for general information and links

Diabetes UK — www.diabetes.org.uk — for information and advice on all aspects of diabetes

European Men's Health Forum — an independent, non-governmental, non-profit-making organisation established to promote male health across Europe — www.emhf.org/index.cfm/item_id/99/

Faith and Food — provides information on what, why and where individuals can eat in accordance with their faith — www.faithandfood.com/

Five-a-day Programme — www.doh.gov.uk/fiveaday

Food and Drink Federation — www.foodfitness.org.uk

Man Health Magazine is an online magazine that provides information on aspects of men's health based on clinical research and real-world experience — www.man-health-magazine-online.com/

Men's Health Forum Ireland seeks to promote, influence and enhance all aspects of the health and well-being of men and boys in Ireland — www.mhfi.org/

National Obesity Forum — www.nationalobesityforum.org.uk

Peak Performance Online — www.pponline.co.uk

SimplyFood — www.simplyfood.com — for food, nutrition and healthy-eating information

Men's Health Forum (Scotland) exists to support the many committed individuals working within the Health Service and the voluntary sector in their efforts, to help men take a more active interest in their health, and to assist service providers to support and encourage men to do so — www.mhfs.org.uk

The Men's Project (Northern Ireland) aims to increase awareness of the issues facing men and boys and promotes their social inclusion — www.mensproject.org

Health For Men (UK) focuses on some of the health issues to which men are particularly susceptible — www.healthformen.co.uk

References

Adolfsson B, Andersson I, Elofsson S, Rossner S, Unden AL (2005) Locus of control and weight reduction. *Patient Educ Couns* **56**: 55–61

APHO (2005) Indications of Public Health in English Regions: Lifestyle and its Impact on Health. Association of Public Health Observatories. http://www.empho.org.uk/sepho_lifestyle_200105.pdf (last accessed February 2005)

Baker P (2001) The state of men's health. *Men's Health J* **1**(1): 6–7

Bandolier (undated) Starting to Exercise. www.jr2.ox.ac.uk/badolier/booth/hliving/startoex.html (last accessed February 2005)

Batty GD, Shiplet MJ, Marmot M, Smith GD (2002) Physical activity and cause-specific mortality in men with type II diabetes/impaired glucose tolerance: evidence from the Whitehall study. *Diabet Med* **19**: 580–88

British Heart Foundation (2004) BHF Coronary Heart Disease Statistics 2004. http://www.bhf.org.uk/professionals/index.asp?SecID=15&secondlevel=519 (last accessed February 2005)

BUPA (2003) Diabetes (Type 2). http://hcd2.bupa.co.uk/fact_sheets/html/diabetes2.html (last accessed February 2005)

Burden M (2003) Diabetes: signs, symptoms and making a diagnosis. *Nurs Times* **99**(1): 30–2

Cale L, Harris J (2001) Exercise recommendations for young people: an update. *Health Educ* **101**(3): 126–38

Cancer Research UK (2005) Alarming ignorance of cancer risk. http://science.cancerresearchuk.org/news/archivednews/redrisk?version=1 (last accessed February 2005)

Caroli M, Lagravinese D (2002) Prevention of obesity. *Nutr Res* **22**: 221–6

Coronary Heart Disease (2000) Guidance for implementing the preventative aspects of the National Service Framework http://www.hda-online.org.uk/downloads/pdfs/chdframework.pdf (last accessed February 2005)

Crawford D (2002) Population strategies to prevent obesity. *BMJ* **325**: 728–9

DoH (1999a) *Reducing Health Inequalities: An Action Report.* London: DoH

DoH (1999b) *Health Survey for England.* London: DoH

DoH (2001) National Service Framework Diabetes: Standards. London: DoH. www.doh.gov.uk/nsf/diabetes (last accessed February 2005)

DoH (2004a) *Choosing Health. Making Healthier Choices Easier.* London: Stationary Office

DoH (2004b) *Choosing Health? Choosing Activity: A Consultation on How to Increase Physical Activity.* London: DoH

DoH Physical Activity, Health Improvement and Prevention (2004) Chapter 3: Recommendations for Active Living throughout the Life Course. In: *At Least Five a Week: Evidence on the Impact of Physical Activity and its Relationship to Health.* London: DoH

Drummond S (2002) The management of obesity. *Nurs Standard* **16**(48): 47–52

Dyer O (2002) First cases of type II diabetes found in white UK teenagers. *BMJ* **324**: 506

Exercise Alliance (2001) Physical Activity — Benefits to Health. http://www.exercisealliance.org.uk/aboutpa/benefits.htm (accessed February 2005)

Gillman MW, Pinto BM, Tennstedt S, Glanz K, Marcus B, Friedman RH (2001) Relationships of physical activity and dietary behaviors among adults. *Prev Med* **32**: 295–301

Hall EE, Ekkekakis P, Petruzzello SJ (2002) The affective beneficence of vigorous exercise revisited. *Br J Health Psychol* **7**: 47–66

Harvey EL, Glenny A–M, Kirk SFL, Summerbell CD (2002) An updated systematic review of interventions to improve health professionals' management of obesity. *Obes Rev* **3**: 45–55

Hughes J, Martin S (1999) The Department of Health's project to evaluate weight management services. *J Hum Nutr Diet* **12**: 1–8

Hunt K, Ford G, Mutrie N (2001) Is sport for all?: exercise and physical activity patterns in early and late middle age in the West of Scotland. *Health Educ* **101**(4): 151–8

Hussey J, Gormley J, Bell C (2001) Physical activity in Dublin children aged 7–9 years. *Br J Sports Med* **35**: 268–73

ICN (2002) ICN on Obesity: Creating Public Awareness of a Social-Environmental Disease. http://www.icn.ch/matters_obesity.htm (last accessed February 2005)

Inchley J, Todd J, Bryce C, Currie C (2001) Dietary trends among Scottish schoolchildren in the 1990s. *Journal of Hum Nutr Dietet* **14**: 207–16

Kennedy LA (2001) Community involvement at what cost? — local appraisal of a pan-European nutrition promotion programme in low-income neighbourhoods. *Health Promot Int* **16**(1): 35–45

Koch T, Kralik D, Taylor J (2000) Men living with diabetes: minimizing the intrusiveness of the disease. *J Clin Nurs* **9**: 247–54

McWhirter L (2002) *Health and Social Care in Northern Ireland: A Statistical Profile*. DoH: Social Care and Public Safety

Melin I, Rossner S (2003) Practical clinical behavioural treatment of obesity. *Patient Educ Counsel* **49**: 75–83

Narayan KMV, Bowman BA, Engelgau ME (2001) Prevention of type II diabetes. *BMJ* **323**: 63

National Audit Office (2001) Tackling Obesity in England. London: HMSO

NHS Scotland (2005) *Scottish Diabetes Framework*. Edinburgh: Scottish Executive

NICE (2004) Final Scope: Obesity. http://www.nice.org.uk/pdf/Obesity_scope_final.pdf (last accessed February 2005)

Noel PH, Pugh JA (2002) Management of overweight and obese adults. *BMJ* **325**: 757–61

Office for National Statistics (2000) *Social Trends 30*. London: HMSO

Parliamentary Office of Science and Technology (POST) (2001) Health benefits of physical activity. http://www.parliament.uk/post/pn162.pdf (last accessed February 2005)

POST (2003) Childhood obesity. http://www.parliament.uk/post/pn205.pdf (last accessed January 2005)

Parmenter K (2002) Changes in nutrition knowledge and dietary behaviour. *Health Educ* **102**(1): 23–9

Parmenter K, Waller J, Wardle J (2000) Demographic variation in nutrition knowledge in England. *Health Educ Res* **15**(2): 163–74

Parry-Langdon N, Roberts C (2004) *Physical Activity, Sedentary Behaviour and Obesity/Gweithgarwch Corfforol, Ymddygiad Eisteddog a Gordewdra*. HBSC Briefing Series: 1. Cardiff: Welsh Assembly Government

Plonczynski DJ (2000) Measurement of motivation for exercise. *Health Educ Res* **15**(6): 695–705

Povey R, Conner M, Sparks P, James R, Shepherd R (2000) Application of the theory of planned behaviour to two dietary behaviours: roles of perceived control and self-efficacy. *Br J Health Psychol* **5**: 121–39

Satia-Abouta J, Patterson RE, Schiller RN, Kristal AR (2002) Energy from far is associated with obesity in U.S. men: results from the prostate cancer prevention trial. *Prev Med* **34**: 493–501

Scottish Executive (2003) Let's Make Scotland More Active: A Strategy for Physical Activity — a Consultation. Physical Activity Taskforce. http://www.scotland.gov. uk/library5/culture/lmsa-00.asp (accessed February 2005)

Scottish Office (1996) *Eating for Health: A Diet Action Plan for Scotland.* Edinburgh: HMSO

Sky News Online (2003) Figures put on effect of weight. *Sky News Online* 07/01/03

Sparling PB, Owen N, Lambert EV, Haskell WL (2000) Promoting physical activity: the new imperative for public health. *Health Educ Res* **15**(3): 367–76

Tanasescu M, Leitzman MF, Rimm EB, Willett WC, Stampfer MJ, Hu FB (2002) Exercise type and intensity in relation to coronary heart disease in men. *JAMA* **288**(16): 1994–2000

Van der Biji AK, Laurant MGH, Wensing M (2002) Effectiveness of physical activity interventions for older adults. *Am J Prev Med* **22**(2): 120–33

Vuori I (1998) Does physical activity enhance health? *Patient Educ Counsel* **33**: S95–S103

West P, Reeder AI, Milne BJ, Poulton R (2002) Worlds apart: a comparison between physical activities among youth in Glasgow, Scotland and Dunedin, New Zealand. *Soc Sci Med* **54**: 607–19

Whelton SP, Chin A, Xin X, He J (2002) Review: aerobic exercise reduced systolic and diastolic blood pressure in adults. *Evid Based Med* **6**: 170

WHO (2002) *Reducing Risks and Promoting Healthy Life.* Geneva: WHO

WHO (2003a) Obesity and Overweight. http://www.who.int/hpr/NPH/docs/gs_ obesity.pdf (last accessed January 2005)

WHO (2003b) Diet, Nutrition and the Prevention of Chronic Diseases. http://www.who.int/nut/documents/trs_916.pdf (accessed February 2005)

Woolf-May K, Kearney EM, Owen A, Jones DW, Davison RCR, Bird SR (1999) The efficacy of accumulated short bouts versus single daily bouts of brisk walking in improving aerobic fitness and blood lipids profiles. *Health Educ Res* **14**(6): 803–15

Chapter 6

Maintaining mental health

An individual's sense of mental health is not separate from their social interaction and sense of self-worth or identity. It affects how they negotiate in the social world and how they form social relationships... Negative regard by others can easily be incorporated by the individual into negative regard of self.

Robertson (1998: 33)

About one fifth of the world's youth suffer from mild to severe mental health disorders.

ICN (2001)

Mental health problems are common and diverse. One in four people will experience a mental health problem at some time in their lives, most commonly anxiety and depression. It is also estimated that one person in every 250 will have a psychotic illness such as schizophrenia or bipolar affective disorder (manic depression). Not everyone with a mental health problem has a severe illness or will experience severe symptoms all of the time and 90% of mental health problems are treated in primary care.

(CHI, 2003)

Mental health

Mental health is about how we think and feel about ourselves and others and how we interpret the world around us. It affects our capacity to cope with change and major life events such as having a baby or experiencing bereavement; it affects our ability to communicate and to form and sustain relationships. Mental health is central to our health and well-being.

National Institute for Mental Health in England (2004a)

Impact of mental health problems

⌘ Only 24% of those with long-term mental health problems are employed.

⌘ People with mental health problems are twice as likely to lose their jobs as those without.

⌘ The first episode of a mental health problem often occurs between the late teens and early twenties.

⌘ Sixty-six per cent of men with health problems who are unemployed and under the age of thirty-five die by suicide.

⌘ People with mental health problems are almost three times more likely to be in financial debt than those without a mental health problem.

⌘ One in four tenants with mental health problems has serious rent arrears and is at risk of losing their home.

⌘ People with severe mental health problems are three times more likely to be divorced than those without a mental health problem.

Source: Office of the Deputy Prime Minister (2004)

Impact of mental health on physical health

⌘ Depression increases the risk of coronary heart disease (CHD) fourfold, even when other risk factors such as smoking are controlled for.

⌘ Depression is a risk factor for stroke.

⌘ Depression has a significant impact on health outcomes for a wide range of chronic physical illnesses, including asthma, arthritis and diabetes.

⌘ Lack of control at work is associated with increased risk of cardiovascular disease.

⌘ Perceived low-control beliefs (powerlessness, fatalism) accounted for more than half the raised mortality risk for people of low socioeconomic status.

⌘ Sustained stress or trauma increases susceptibility to viral infection and physical illness by damaging the immune system.

⌘ Emotional well-being is a strong predictor of physical health.

Source: DoH (2001a)

Factors that have a positive impact on mental health are: good support networks; good general health; leisure time; a social life; and a good income. Conversely, factors that have a negative impact on mental health are: stress; poor general health; and lack of money (Glendinning *et al*, 2002).

Mental health promotion

Mental health promotion involves any action to enhance the mental well-being of individuals, families, organisations or communities. It is about strengthening protective factors and reducing risk factors for mental health... It recognises that how people feel is a significant influence on health.

(National Institute for Mental Health in England 2004a)

According to the National Institute for Mental Health in England (2004a: 3), 'mental health promotion operates at three interconnected levels:

⌘ **Strengthening individuals**: increasing emotional resilience by promoting self-esteem, life and coping skills (for example, communicating, negotiating, relationship and parenting skills) and enabling people from different black and minority ethnic populations to develop a positive cultural identity and thereby build their confidence and sense of worth.

⌘ **Strengthening communities**: increasing social support, social inclusion and participation, improving community safety, neighbourhood environments, promoting childcare and self-help networks, promoting mental health within schools and workplaces eg. through anti-bullying strategies and race-equality schemes, programmes to tackle racism within schools, workplaces and the wider community.

⌘ **Reducing structural barriers to mental health**: challenging stereotypes, discrimination and inequalities and reducing the political, social and economic barriers influencing the capacity of different black and minority ethnic groups to participate. Work to develop health and social services that support and promote mental health; ensure people have good access to good-quality health care; increase access to education, meaningful employment, training opportunities, housing, benefit entitlements and support for vulnerable people.'

In its document *Making It Happen* (2001a), the DoH presents two tables, reproduced from Australia's National Mental Health Strategy (2000), which summarise protective and risk factors for the development of mental health problems and disorders at different levels and in different settings:

Box 6.1: Protective factors against the development of mental health problems and disorders

❖ *Individual factors*: easy temperament; adequate nutrition; attachment to family; above-average intelligence; school achievement; problem-solving skills; internal locus of control; social competence/skills; good coping style; optimism; moral beliefs/values; positive self-image.

❖ *Family factors*: supportive caring parent(s); family harmony; secure and stable family; small family size; more than two years between siblings; responsibility within the family (for child or adult);supportive relationship with an adult (for child or adult); strong family norms and morality.

❖ *School context*: sense of belonging; positive school climate; prosocial peer group; required responsibility and helpfulness; opportunities for some success and recognition of achievements; school norms against violence.

❖ *Life events and situations*: involvement with 'significant other' (partner/mentor); availability of opportunities at critical turning points or major transitions; economic security; good physical health.

❖ *Community and cultural factors*: sense of 'connectedness'; attachments to, and networks within, the community; participation in Church or other community group; strong cultural identity and ethnic pride; access to support services; community/cultural norms against violence.

Box 6.2: Risk factors for the development of mental health problems and disorders

❖ *Individual factors*: prenatal brain damage; prematurity; birth injury; low birth weight; birth complications; physical and intellectual disability; poor health in infancy; insecure attachment in infant/child; low intelligence; difficult temperament; chronic illness; poor social skills; low self-esteem; alienation; impulsivity.

❖ *Family factors*: having a teenage mother; having a lone parent;absence
  of father in childhood; large family size; anti-social role models (in
  childhood); family violence and disharmony; marital discord in parents;
  poor supervision and monitoring of child; low parental involvement
  in child's activities; neglect in childhood; long-term parental
  unemployment; criminality in parent; parental substance abuse; parental
  mental disorder; harsh or inconsistent discipline style; social isolation;
  experience of rejection; lack of warmth and affection.
❖ *School context*: bullying; peer rejection; poor attachment to school;
  inadequate behaviour management; deviant peer group; school failure.
❖ *Life events and situations*: physical, sexual and emotional abuse;
  school transitions; divorce and family break-up; death of family
  member; physical illness/impairment; unemployment; homelessness;
  incarceration; poverty/economic insecurity; job insecurity; unsatisfactory
  workplace relationships; workplace accident/injury; caring for someone
  with an illness/disability; living in a nursing home or aged care hostel;
  war or natural disasters.
❖ *Community and cultural factors*: socioeconomic disadvantage; social
  or cultural discrimination; isolation; neighbourhood violence and crime;
  population density and housing conditions; lack of support service
  including transport, shopping, recreational facilities.

Stress

*Stress is what happens when the pressure you are under is more than
you think you can cope with.*

Samaritans with Cary Cooper (2001)

*Stress is the natural reaction people have to excessive pressures or
other types of demand placed on them.*

Health and Safety Executive (2000)

The following quotation describes the link between physical and mental
health.

*We are now beginning to recognise that people's social and
psychological circumstances can seriously damage their health in
the long term. Chronic anxiety, insecurity, low self esteem, social
isolation and lack of control over work appear to undermine mental*

*and physical health. The power of psycho-social factors to affect
health makes biological sense. The human body has evolved to
response automatically to emergencies. This stress response activates
a cascade of stress hormones, which affects the cardio-vascular, and
immune systems. The rapid reaction of our hormones and nervous
systems. The rapid reaction of our hormones and nervous system
prepares the individual to deal with a brief physical threat. But
if the biological stress response is activated too often and for too
long, there may be multiple health costs. These include depression,
increased susceptibility to infection, diabetes, high blood pressure
and accumulation of cholesterol in blood vessel walls, with the
attendant risks of heart attack and stroke.*

Brunner and Marmot (1999: 41)

The BHF (2004) offer the following twenty-three item checklist of possible symptoms of stress. They state that if someone ticks five or more of the following items, they may be suffering from stress:

- feeling sweaty or shivery
- pounding heart or palpitations
- needing to go to the toilet a lot more than normal
- feeling sick in the stomach ('having butterflies')
- dry mouth
- exhaustion
- odd aches and pains
- smoking and drinking more
- working to exhaustion
- headaches
- no time for hobbies any more
- being irritable at everything
- thinking 'I can't cope with this any more'
- loss of appetite for food, fun or sex
- eating too much or too little
- loss of sense of humour
- loss of interest in personal appearance
- loss of interest in other people
- a feeling that everything is pointless
- tearfulness
- forgetfulness
- feeling tired and having no energy
- difficulty in sleeping, disturbed sleep and waking up unusually early

Work-related stress

Work-related stress affects about one in five workers (approximately five million people).

DoH (2001a)

Work-related stress is 'the adverse reaction people have to excessive pressure or other types of demand placed on them. Pressure is part and parcel of all work and helps to keep us motivated. But excessive pressure can lead to stress which undermines performance, is costly to employers, and can make people ill'.

Health and Safety Executive (2004)

De Vries *et al* (2003) state that the following factors can lead to work-related stress:

⌘   Unreasonably long hours.
⌘   Work overload or underload.
⌘   Role ambiguity, role conflict and unclear mandates.
⌘   Undefined but (somehow) important work relationships that contribute little but distraction.
⌘   Poor communication up and down the workplace hierarchy and laterally among peers.
⌘   Job insecurity intensified by unresponsive managers; mistrust; over-promotion; vicious office politics; and imbalance between life and work obligations.

Wilkerson (2002) adds doubt, feeling unappreciated and inconsistent management processes to the factors above.

White (2001) notes that high demands and low control at work are associated with psychological distress and health complaints. Hemingway and Marmot (1999) assert that having control over one's work is more significant than either the pace or variety of tasks. BHF (2002) suggests that about 33% of men experience a high pace of work. Thirty-one percent of women reported that they experienced low control compared with 19% of men. Men in Social Class V were eight times more likely to report a lack of control over their work than those in Social Class I.

Kivimaki *et al* (2002) carried out a prospective cohort study of 812 Finnish men who were in work. Their aim was to examine the association between work stress and the risk of death from cardiovascular disease. They found a two-fold higher cardiovascular mortality risk among people with high job strain and an imbalance in reward for effort.

Box 6.3: Key facts about work-related stress

⌘ About 500,000 people in the UK believe that they experience work-related stress to an extent that makes them ill.

⌘ About 500,000 people in the UK felt 'extremely' or 'very' stressed by their work.

⌘ Work-related stress is thought to lose the EU at least 20 billion per year in time and health costs. In the UK, the annual figure is estimated to be around £3.7 billion.

⌘ Twenty-eight per cent of employees in the EU report that they are affected by work-related stress.

⌘ Women appear to suffer slightly more than men.

⌘ Common causes include lack of job security and control, and work overload.

⌘ Over 50% of absenteeism has its roots in work-related stress.

⌘ The human costs of stress are significant. It is estimated that 16% of male and 22% of female cardiovascular disease in the EU is due towork-related stress.

Sources: Health and Safety Authority (2002); Health and Safety Executive (2004a)

The DoH (2001a) reports the findings from two relevant research studies. First, the Whitehall II study found that an imbalance between effort and reward increased the risk of alcohol dependence in men by 70–90% and that psychological demands, work overload, low social support and an imbalance between effort and reward were associated with an increased risk of psychiatric disorder in both men and women. Second, the DoH (2001a) document refers to the findings by the Health and Safety Executive, which show that: there is a link between design of jobs and levels of stress; that stress has an impact on physical and mental health, including back pain, drinking and smoking; that low levels of job control are associated with poor mental health in men and increased risk of alcohol dependence in women; and that feeling unsupported increases the risk of psychiatric problems.

The Health and Safety Executive (2004b) highlights that work-related stressorsare culture; demands of the job; control; relationships; change; role and support; and the individual. It presents the following information:

Culture

❖ Problems that can lead to stress:

- lack of communication and consultation.
- a culture of blame when things go wrong; denial of potential problems.
- an expectation that people will regularly work excessively long hours or take work home with them.

❖ What management can do:

- provide opportunities for staff to contribute ideas, especially in planning and organising their own jobs.
- introduce clear business objectives, good communication and close employee involvement, particularly during periods of change.
- be honest with yourself, set a good example, and listen to and respect others.
- be approachable — create an atmosphere in which people feel it is acceptable to talk to you about any problems they are having.
- avoid encouraging people to work excessively long hours.

Demands of the job

❖ Problems that can lead to stress:

- too much to do in too little time.
- too little or too much training for the job.
- boring or repetitive work or too little to do.
- difficult working environment.

❖ What management can do:

- prioritise tasks; cut out unnecessary work; try to give warning of urgent or important jobs.
- make sure individuals are matched to jobs; provide training for those who need more; increase the scope of jobs for those who are over-trained.
- change the way jobs are done by moving people between jobs, giving individuals more responsibility and increasing

the scope of the job; increasing the variety of tasks, giving
a group of workers greater responsibility for effective
performance of the group.
● make sure workplace hazards such as noise, harmful
substances and the threat of violence are properly controlled.

Control

❖ Problems that can lead to stress:

● lack of control over work activities.

❖ What management can do:

● give more control to staff by enabling them to plan their
own work and make decisions about how that work should be
completed, and how problems should be tackled.

Role

❖ Problems that can lead to stress:

● staff feeling that the job requires them to behave in
conflicting ways at the same time.
● confusion about how everyone fits in.

❖ What management can do:

● talk to people regularly to make sure that everyone is clear
about what their job requires them to do.
● make sure that everyone has clearly defined objectives and
responsibilities linked to business objectives and training on
how everyone fits in.

Relationships

❖ Problems that can lead to stress:

● poor relationships with others.

- bullying; racial or sexual harassment.

❖ What management can do:

- provide training in interpersonal skill.
- set up effective systems to prevent bullying and harassment (ie. a policy, an agreed grievance procedure, and a proper investigation of complaints).

Change

❖ Problems that can lead to stress:

- uncertainty about what is happening.
- fears about job security.

❖ What management can do:

- ensure good communication with staff.
- provide effective support for staff throughout the process.

Support and the individual

❖ Problems that can lead to stress:

- lack of support from managers and co-workers.
- not being able to balance the demands of work and life outside the work setting.

❖ What management can do:

- support and encourage staff, even when things go wrong.
- encourage a healthy work-life balance.
- see if there is scope for flexible work schedules (eg. flexible working hours, working from home, etc).
- take into account that everyone is different and try to allocate work so that everyone is working in the best way that helps them work best.

Preventing work-related stress

In another related publication, the Health and Safety Executive (2004a) and the BHF (2004) suggest the following activities that individuals can follow:

⌘ Eat healthily rather than eating 'on the run' or at one's desk.

⌘ Stop smoking.

⌘ Try to keep within Government recommendations for alcohol consumption — alcohol acts as a depressant and will not help you.

⌘ Watch your caffeine intake — tea, coffee and some soft drinks (eg. cola drinks) may contribute to making you feel more anxious.

⌘ Be physically active — it stimulates you and gives you more energy. But avoid rushing about trying to be available to everybody.

⌘ Avoid trying to do several jobs at once.

⌘ Make time for exercise and relaxation. Try learning relaxation techniques — some people find it helps them cope with pressures in the short term.

⌘ Avoid taking work home with you, if possible.

⌘ Seek help or information — for example, about time management, stress management, or assertiveness training.

⌘ Talk to family, friends or work colleagues about what you are feeling — they may be able to help you and provide the support you need to raise your concerns at work.

⌘ Find out about joining a support group or getting counselling.

⌘ Learn to say 'no' when over-burdened.

Mental health problems

One in six adults has a mental health problem such as anxiety or depression

Wanless (2002)

Mental health is crucial to the well-being of individuals, societies and countries... [it] is more than the absence of mental disorders. It involves a state of well-being whereby the individual recognises their abilities, is able to cope with the normal stresses of life, works productively and contributes to the community.

International Council of Nursing

Men and seeking help

It is well-documented that whilst women are more likely to be diagnosed with depression and anxiety, men are four times more likely than women to commit suicide (DoH, 2001a). The reason for these differences has been the subject of research for many years. The manner by which men are socialised has a direct bearing on their reluctance to seek help (see *Chapter 1*). Ritchie (1999) did a qualitative study whose aim was to understand the barriers that young men perceived as preventing them using support in a crisis. With a sample of eighteen men between the ages of sixteen and thirty-five, she conducted a range of focus groups, using vignettes. Ritchie found that men in all the focus groups equated emotional health with control and discipline. This finding parallels the social norm of what is expected of masculine behaviour.

Emotional health is defined by Ewles and Simnett (2003) as 'the ability to recognise such emotions as fear, joy, grief and anger and to express emotions appropriately.' However, it is recognised that men have difficulty expressing many of these emotions. In Ritchie's (1999) research, she found that men perceived asking for help in a crisis as being the last resort. Young men saw the sharing of feelings and self-disclosure as a taboo because such behaviour went against the male norm. Luck *et al* (2000) argue that because of how they are socialised, men learn to hide their emotions by channelling them in other ways. For example, playing sport or being a spectator; using sex as an outlet; depending on women to fulfill their emotional needs; and assuming that alcohol or drugs permit and enhance the expression of emotions. Ritchie (1999) found that young men viewed alcohol as a way to mask their feelings and that it was often used as a means of coping.

Lloyd and Forrest (2001) state that young men are three times more likely than young women to be alcohol-dependent, and twice as likely to be drug-dependent. Individuals between the ages of twenty and twenty-four are believed to be at particular risk.

Alexander (2001) also carried out a qualitative research study using a sample of eighteen men with the aim of investigating the close relationships of depressed men. Reinforcing Ritchie's (1999) findings, Alexander found that men viewed asking for help as expressions of weakness and dependency. On further investigation, Alexander found that men in the study reported that the way in which they are socialised makes them intolerant of anyone showing weakness or dependency. This, in turn, argues Alexander, makes men intolerant of depression, as they see it as an expression of weakness and emotion, which are normally attributed to women. Courtenay (2000) expands on this by pointing out that since depression is often associated with feelings of powerlessness and lack of control, men construe depression as a sign of failure. It is therefore not surprising that men who have signs of depression present themselves to their GP complaining of physical symptoms.

In a qualitative study that aimed to investigate patients' perceptions of how much time would be afforded them in general-practice consultations for depression, Pollock and Grime (2002) found that 'patients with depression feel under such acute pressure of time that they are often inhibited from fully disclosing their problems, preventing them making the best use of the consulation.' Courtenay (2000) also observes that clinicians were less likely to identify the presence of depression in men than in women, and that they failed to diagnose nearly 65% of depressed men.

Courtenay (2000) asserts that men are much more likely than women to rely on themselves or 'go it alone' to deal with their depression. He reports that, nationally, nearly 50% of men over forty-nine years who reported experiencing depression did not discuss it with anyone, preferring to withdraw socially and deal with it individually by using alcohol or drugs to distract themselves or alleviate their depression. Elgie (2002) confirms that resorting to alcohol, illicit drugs and substance abuse is commonly the way men cope with depression (*Box 6.4, opposite*).

Stigma

Mental illness stigma refers to the negative attitudes held about people with mental health problems.

de Vries *et al* (2003: 45)

Due to stigmatisation of those with mental illness, men are even less likely to ask for help from the mental health services.

Lloyd and Forrest (2001: 36)

For me stigma means fear, resulting in a lack of confidence. Stigma is loss, resulting in unresolved mourning issues. Stigma is not having access to resources... Stigma is being invisible or being reviled, resulting in conflict. Stigma is lowered family esteem and intense shame, resulting in decreased self-worth. Stigma is secrecy... Stigma is anger, resulting in distance. Most importantly, stigma is hopelessness, resulting in helplessness.

(Byrne, 2000: 66)

Box 6.4: Key facts about mental health problems

⌘ About one-fifth of the world's youth suffer from mild to severe mental health problems.

⌘ 400 million people in the world suffer from mental or behavioural disorders.

⌘ Severe mental health problems such as schizophrenia are comparatively rare (schizophrenia occurs in one in 200 adults every year).

⌘ In Europe, one in four men will be affected by a mental illness in their lifetime.

⌘ In England, 14% of men have some form of mental health illness.

⌘ At any one time in the UK, one in six of the population can be affected by depression, anxiety or a phobia. The highest rates are found in deprived areas.

⌘ One third of GPs' time is estimated to focus on patients with mental health problems.

⌘ In Scotland, depression and affective disorders are amongst the commonest reasons for visiting a GP and the commonest reason for those aged between twenty-five and forty-four.

⌘ Mental health problems are estimated to cost the UK over £77 billion a year.

⌘ Sixty-nine per cent of patients with mental disorders usually present to physicians with physical symptoms and many of then are often not correctly treated.

⌘ Around 25% of the total drug bill in the UK can be attributed to drugs for treating mental problems.

⌘ Widowers living alone after the death of their wife appear to be at greater risk of depression.

⌘ There is a link between physical health and mental health. Depression, for example, is linked to mortality following a heart attack; it increases the risk of heart disease by four even when the added risk of smoking is taken into account.

Sources: European Men's Health Forum (www.emhf.org); www.mindout.clarity. uk.net; ICN (2001); Mental Health Foundation (2003); Braunholz *et al* (2004); Choosing Health (2004); ODPM (2004a).

Unlike most people suffering from a physical illness, individuals suffering from a mental health problem are subjected to stigma, prejudice and exclusion (ICN, 2001). Stigma is often due to public ignorance (ICN, 2001), but an increase in knowledge of mental illness alone does not necessarily reduce stigma (DoH, 2001a). The challenge is to reduce stigma associated with mental illness so that individuals will feel more able to express themselves.

Gelder (2001) carried out an opinion poll with the aim of discovering the extent to which the general public attached stigma towards six types of mental illness. The random sample of 1737 people revealed the following findings:

- stigmatising mental health conditions was common
- more than 66% of the sample believed that people with schizophrenia and those with drug addition were dangerous to others. About 75% of people with schizophrenia thought that others perceived them as dangerous
- about 75% believed that people with schizophrenia and substance abuse were unpredictable
- around 50% believed that people with severe depression, dementia and panic attacks were unpredictable
- about 60% of the sample stated they would find it difficult to speak to people who had schizophrenia or depression or abused substances. About 50% of people with schizophrenia thought that others found it difficult to talk to them
- people with alcohol or drug addiction are stigmatised more than those with schizophrenia.

The charity Mind out for Mental Health (http://mindout.clarity.uk.net/) state that in relation to discriminatory practices against people with mental health problems:

- thirty-four per cent felt they had been dismissed or forced to resign from their employment
- sixty-nine per cent were frightened to apply for a job because of anticipated discrimination
- forty-seven per cent had been abused or harassed in public and 14% had been physically abused
- twenty-one per centhad been attacked or harassed by their neighbours
- seventy-three per centbelieved that the way in which mental illness was portrayed by the media was unfair, unbalanced or very negative.

Myths about mental health problems

Table 6.1: Myths and reality about mental health problems	
Myth	**Reality**
People with mental health problems are dangerous and violent	People with a mental health problem are much more likely to be the victim of violence rather than the perpetrator
Mental health problems are rare	During their lifetime, almost everyone will know of someone who has experienced a mental health problem
People with mental health problems are incapable of work	Research from the USA shows that about 58% of people with severe mental health problems can continue to work productively with the correct type of support
People with mental health problems do not want to work	35% of people with mental health problems who are unemployed would like to be able to earn a living, compared with 28% of those with other health conditions

Source: ODPM (2004b)

Risk factors for developing mental health problems

⌘ Unemployment: being unemployed means a loss in status, purpose, social contacts and time-structure to the day, as well as financial loss (Coleman and Hendry, 1999). Unemployed people are twice as likely to have depression as people in work (DoH, 1999). Unemployed men are twice as likely as employed men to commit suicide (Davidson and Lloyd, 2001).

⌘ Bereavement (DoH, 2001b) and anniversary of death (Goldney, 2002).

⌘ Family history of psychiatric disorder (DoH, 2001b; Goldney, 2002).

⌘ Violence (DoH, 2001b). People who have been abused or been victims of domestic violence have higher rates of mental health problems (DoH, 1999).

⌘ Childhood neglect (DoH, 2001b).

⌘ Financial strain (DoH, 2001b). Those who are unemployed are almost twice as likely to show signs of a possible mental health problem. People who have experienced major financial difficulties in the past twelve months are three times more likely to show signs of a possible mental health problem. Children in the poorest households are three times more likely to have mental health problems than children in well-off households (DoH, 1999).

⌘ Family breakdown (DoH, 2001b). Those people who are separated or divorced from their partner are more likely to show signs of a possible mental health problem.

⌘ Being in long-term care (DoH, 2001b; Goldney, 2002).

⌘ Homelessness: between a quarter and a half of people using night shelters or sleeping rough may have a serious mental disorder; up to about half may be alcohol-dependent (DoH, 1999).

⌘ Ethnicity: some black and minority ethnic groups are diagnosed as having higher rates of mental disorder than the general population; refugees and migrants are especially vulnerable (DoH 1999; Goldney 2002).

⌘ Being in prison: there is a high rate of mental disorder in the prison population (DoH, 1999).

⌘ Drug and alcohol problems: people with drug and alcohol problems have higher rates of other mental health problems (DoH, 1999; Goldney, 2002).

⌘ Having sexual-identity conflicts (Goldney, 2002).

⌘ Having debilitating physical illness (Goldney, 2002).

Depression

Depression will be one of the largest problems worldwide by 2020.

Herrman (2001: 710)

Every week, 10% of the UK population aged sixteen to sixty-five report significant depressive symptoms and one in ten of these admits to suicidal thinking.

Davies *et al* (2001: 1500)

Depression is a serious and common mental illness. It is a feeling of constant sadness. It affects sleep, appetite and concentration. Approximately six million people suffer from depression in the UK. It is predicted that by 2020 depression will be the second leading cause of disease burden. Up to 50% of people with clinical depression do not receive proper diagnosis and treatment for their illness.

www.emental-health.com/depr_fastfacts.htm (accessed January 2005)

Depression can affect anyone, male or female, at any age, and almost at any time. It is not feeling 'blue' or 'down' for a couple of days, but is a longer-lasting condition that can dominate daily life. Each year, one in fifteen women and one in thirty men will be affected by depression and every GP will see between sixty and 100 people with depression (DoH, 1999). Men who live alone are more prone to depression (Alexander, 2001).

> *Depression is an illness that affects both men and women. But people working in mental health services see far fewer men with depression than women with depression. It seems likely that men suffer depression just as often as women, but that they are less likely to ask for help... Depression causes a huge amount of suffering. It is a major reason for people taking time off sick from their work. Many people who kill themselves have been depressed — it is a potentially fatal disorder. However, it is easily treatable and best treated as early as possible.*
>
> Royal College of Psychiatrists (2002)

It is suggested that if an individual suffers from depression, there is a 50% chance it is due to genetic factors and a 50% chance it is due to environmental factors. The average age for someone to become depressed is under thirty years (www.at-ease.nsf.org.uk/depression(1).html, last accessed February 2005).

In the UK, rates of anxiety and depression are low in Chinese communities whilst there is an over diagnosis of schizophrenia in African Caribbean's and under diagnosis of depression in African Caribbean's and South Asian's (National Institute of Mental Health in England, 2004b).

According to the Royal College of Psychiatrists (2002), the signs and symptoms of depression can be divided into psychological and physical and other aspects that people may notice. Psychological symptoms include feeling unhappy and miserable all the time, which can be worse first thing in the morning. Other symptoms include the inability to enjoy anything or to concentrate properly; and to feel guilty without reason. Physical symptoms include an inability to get to sleep and then waking early and during the night; loss of libido; inability to eat and loss of weight. Other people may notice depressed individuals performing less well at work; being unusually quiet and unable to talk about things; worrying more than usual; being more irritable than usual; and complaining more about vague physical problems.

Males and females differ in the manner in which they express depression. Whilst women tend to talk about and share their feelings, men often exhibit hostility and anger. According to Alexander (2001), the way in which men are socialised causes them to be particularly intolerant of depression because they should be emotionally strong and being depressed makes them be perceived as weak, unstable or unmanly. Sleath and Rubin (2002: 243) report that when patients attend their GP, they 'only give general hints about the presence of emotional distress and share more personal information only when encouraged by the physician'. This is perhaps compounded by the fact that men are more likely to present with physical symptoms or work-related problems rather than symptoms of depression *per se*.

Men who live alone are more prone to depression (Alexander, 2001). According to Gilbody and Whitty (2002), of the 80% of patients who have depression and do not provide any indication to their GP as to the underlying psychological nature of their problem, 50% of these cases are misdiagnosed. Of the estimated 33 million people in Europe who suffer from depression, only 18% are prescribed the correct treatment (White and Cash, 2003).

Risk factors associated with the development of depression

⌘ **Unemployment**: up to one in seven men who become unemployed will develop a depressive illness in the next six months (Royal College of Psychiatrists, 2002). This can be attributed to the loss of work and therefore the loss of sense of self-worth and self-esteem, as well as loss of symbols of achievement such as company car and loss of control over life events. The loss of social networks may also be a contributing factor.
⌘ **Ethnicity**: the rate of depression in African-Caribbeans, Asians, refugees and asylum seekers is 60% higher than in the white population, with the difference twice as great for men (DoH, 1999).
⌘ **Genetics**: there is growing research evidence that individuals may have a genetic predisposition to developing depression. The son or daughter of a manically depressed parent runs a twenty times higher risk than normal of developing the illness (www.sane.org.uk).
⌘ **Physical illness**: there is evidence that a number of physical illnesses or conditions can cause depression. These include: glandular fever; having chemotherapy or radiotherapy; life-threatening or mutilating surgery; Parkinson's disease; multiple sclerosis; stroke; epilepsy; malnutrition; and drinking excessive amounts of alcohol (www.sane.org.uk).
⌘ **Social factors**: unemployment; bereavement; divorce; rejection as an adult or in childhood; social isolation (www.sane.org.uk).

Self-help when depressed

⌘ Don't bottle things up — try to share how you feel with others.
⌘ Keep active — this will keep you physically fit and you'll sleep better.
⌘ Eat properly — it's easy to lose weight and run low on vitamins when you're depressed.
⌘ Avoid alcohol and drugs — alcohol may make you feel better in the short term, but in the longer term it makes you more depressed. The same goes

for street drugs, particularly amphetamines and ecstasy.

⌘ Don't get upset if you cannot sleep — do something restful that you enjoy, like listening to the radio or watching television.

⌘ Use relaxation techniques.

⌘ Do something you enjoy — set aside time regularly each week.

⌘ Examine your lifestyle — a lot of people who have depression are perfectionists and drive themselves too hard. You may need to set yourself more realistic targets and reduce your workload.

⌘ Take a break — it can be really helpful to get away and out of your normal routine for a few days. Even a few hours can be helpful.

⌘ Read about depression — this can help you cope, and books can also help friends and relatives to understand what you're going through.

Source: Royal College of Psychiatrists (2002)

Research highlights that physical activity is particularly effective in both preventing and treating mental health problems. Physical activity is known to improve emotions and mood, increase self-esteem and provide a sense of control (Faulkner and Biddle, 1999; 2002).

Deliberate self-harm

Self-harm is really a broad term for many acts which cause personal harm, whether deliberate or not. It can incorporate a wide range of self-abusive patterns. These can range from failure to give attention to one's own emotional or physical needs, right through to more direct forms of self-laceration, burning or injury through taking toxic substances. Self-harm can also include eating disorders and addictive behaviour. It is the equivalent of an expression of an inner scream... it's a non-verbal form of communication in which feelings can be externalised.

Harrison (2000: 2)

According to Coleman and Hendry (1999), deliberate self-harm is the commonest reason for acute medical admission of young people. It is common in adolescents, especially girls. There are estimated to be 25,000 episodes in England and Wales each year (Hawton *et al*, 2002). However, this may be an underestimate, since many individuals hide the fact that they self-harm. Hawton *et al* (2002: 1208) define deliberate self-harm as an 'act with a non-fatal outcome in which an individual deliberately did one or more of the following:

⌘ Initiated behaviour (for example, self-cutting, jumping from a height), which they intended to cause self-harm.

⌘ Ingested a substance in excess of the prescribed or generally recognised therapeutic dose.

⌘ Ingested a recreational or illicit drug that was an act that the person regarded as self-harm.

⌘ Ingested a non-ingestible substance or object.'

In relation to men exhibiting deliberate self-harm, Harrison (2000) notes that men who are incarcerated in prison, particularly if they have a history of abuse, may resort to deliberate self-harm as way of expressing their pent-up feelings. Harrison (2000) usefully differentiates between self-harm and suicide: 'Self-harm provides the means to survive overwhelming emotions — a way to control feelings of helplessness and powerless. Feelings are numbed or killed off in order to survive deeper hopelessness and despair. This is actually quite different from seeking annihilation.'

In their study, which aimed to determine the prevalence of deliberate self-harm in adolescents in schools in England, Hawton *et al* (2002) discovered that the factors associated with self-harm included recent awareness of self-harm in peers or family (possibly a modelling affect); drug misuse; depression; anxiety; impulsivity, and low self-esteem. The rates of deliberate self-harm have increased dramatically over the last twenty years (Repper, 1999). Indeed, Reeper states that it is the second highest cause of admission to medical wards for men after coronary heart disease (CHD).

Faltermeyer and Pryjmachuk (2000) observe that whilst stress manifests itself most commonly in women as anxiety or depression, in men it manifests itself as aggression. The number of men who self-harm is increasing (www. netdoctor.co.uk/menshealth/facts/depressionsuicide.htm). This aggression, according to Faltermeyer and Pryjmachuk, when focused on oneself, leads to deliberate self-harm or suicide. Warm *et al* (2003: 77) carried out a survey of 243 people (205 females and thirty-four males) and found that the 'majority of respondents believed that self-harm is a means of expressing emotional pain and anger and can be used as a form of coping and a way of staying in control.'

Box 6.5: Key facts about self-harm

⌘ The rates of self-harm in the UK are amongst the highest in Europe and have increased in the last ten years.

⌘ Over 24,000 UK teenagers are admitted to hospital after self-harming.

⌘ The average age of the onset of self-harming is thirteen years old.

⌘ The onset of self-harming is often associated with bullying; relationship difficulties; abuse; rape; and bereavement.

Source: http://www.seemescotland.org/facts/index.php
(accessed February 2005)

Drug use, misuse and abuse

In the UK alone, approximately 3.5 million individuals go to nightclubs each week. Most of these are younger people and a large proportion of them consume illegal drugs, often in combination with alcohol.

Bellis *et al* (2002: 1025)

Around four million people use at least one illicit drug each year and around one million people use at least one of the most dangerous drugs (such as ecstasy, heroin and cocaine) classified as Class A. Many of these individuals will take drugs once, but for around 250,000 problematic drug users in England and Wales, drugs cause considerable harm to themselves and others. Drug misuse gives rise to between £10 billion and £18 billion a year in social and economic costs, 99% of which are accounted for by problematic drug users.

Home Office Drugs Strategy Directorate (2002: 8)

The most commonly used illegal drug among eleven to twenty-four year-olds is cannabis (*grass, dope, weed, puff*). Other drugs frequently used are volatile solvents, such as glue and butane gas, ecstasy (*E*), amphetamines (*speed*), LSD (*acid*) and tranquillisers. Heroin (*smack*) and cocaine (*coke, charlie*) are much less frequently used by young people (Royal College of Psychiatrists, 1999b).

Coulthard *et al* (2002) provide the lifetime prevalence rates for the most misused and abused drugs: cannabis (24%); amphetamines (7%); magic mushrooms (5%); ecstasy, cocaine, or LSD (4%); tranquillisers (3%) and glue (1%).

Box 6.6: Key facts about drug-taking among men

⌘ Men are more likely than women to use illegal drugs.
⌘ Men are twice as likely than women to have had an overdose.
⌘ Drug dependence is associated with being in the sixteen to twenty-four age-group; being single; unemployed; in financial difficulties; living in private rented accommodation, as well as being male.

Why do men use drugs?

⌘ To enjoy the short-term effects — the 'highs'.
⌘ To improve work, sport and sexual performance.
⌘ Curiosity.
⌘ Peer-pressure.
⌘ The drugs are 'there' and available.

What are the risks of taking drugs?

⌘ You can't be entirely sure how the drug will affect you, even if you've taken it before.
⌘ You can rarely be sure how pure or strong the drug is, or what it has been mixed with. This means there is a chance that you could overdose.
⌘ Injecting drugs puts you at risk of contracting Hepatitis B, Hepatitis C and HIV, the virus that causes AIDS.

Sources: Coulthard *et al* (2002); Dr Rob Hicks at:
www.bbc.co.uk/health/mens/life_drugs.shtml#report
(last accessed February 2005)

Boreham and Shaw (2001) carried out a survey of smoking, drinking and drug-use among secondary-school pupils (aged eleven to fifteen years) in England and found the following:

⌘ In 2000, nearly nine in ten (88%) of pupils had heard of cannabis; 86% had heard of cocaine; and 85% had heard of heroin.
⌘ Thirty-six per cent had been offered at least one drug at some point: 28% had been offered cannabis; 17% cocaine/ecstasy; and 6% heroin.
⌘ Sixty-one per cent of pupils had been offered drugs by fifteen years of age, and 15% by the age of eleven.

⌘ Among fifteen year-olds, 32% had used drugs; 29% had used drugs in the last year; and 21% had used drugs in the last month.

⌘ By fifteen years of age, three in ten pupils had used at least one drug in the last year, nearly all of whom had used cannabis.

⌘ Pupils who either drank or smoked were more likely to take drugs.

⌘ There is a stronger link between smoking and drug-taking than between smoking and drinking, or between drinking and drug-use.

According to Boys *et al* (2001: 457), it is estimated that 50% of young people between sixteen and twenty-four years-old have used an illicit drug on at least one occasion in their lives: 'Amongst sixteen to nineteen and twenty to twenty-four year-olds, the most prevalent drug is cannabis (used by 40% of sixteen to nineteen year-olds and 47% of twenty to twenty-four year-olds), followed by amphetamine sulphate (18% and 24% of the two age-groups, respectively), LSD (10% and 13%) and ecstasy (8% and 12%). Boys *et al* (2001) did a quantitative study using a sample of 364 young drug-users aged between sixteen and twenty-two years with the aim of discovering the reasons why they used drugs. The reasons cited were using them to relax (96.7%); become intoxicated (96.4%); keep awake at night while socialising (95.9%); enhance an activity (88.5%); and alleviate depressed mood (86.8%). Men are more likely than women to use illegal drugs (*Table 6.1*), which have a range of major health risks (*Table 6.2*).

Table 6.1: Percentage of men in England and Wales (1998) who had used drugs in the past year				
Drug	**Age group (years)**			
	16–24	25–34	35–44	45–59
Cannabis	32%	17%	6%	3%
Amphetamines	12%	5%	1%	—
Poppers	7%	2%	1%	—
Ecstasy	6%	2%	—	—
Cocaine	4%	3%	1%	—
LSD	5%	1%	—	—
Magic mushrooms	5%	1%	—	0
Heroin	1%	—	—	—

Source: http://www.statistics.gov.uk/STATBASE/Expodata/Spreadsheets/D4456.xls
(last accessed February 2005)

Table 6.2: Illegal drugs and their major health risks	
Drug	**Health risk**
Cannabis	Impotence, low sperm count, anxiety, paranoia, depression
Amphetamines	Anxiety, panic attacks, hallucinations, heart damage with long-term use
Ecstasy	Over-heating and dehydration from over-exertion, liver and kidney problems, possible brain damage
Cocaine	Fatal heart problems, convulsions, depression
Heroin	Breathing problems, risks of injection: vein damage, hepatitis B and C, HIV
Gases, glues, aerosols	Black-outs, fatal heart problems, brain damage

Source: Rob Hicks: www.bbc.co.uk/health/mens/life_drugs.shtml#report
(accessed February 2005)

Drug misuse is related to risk factors such as those that increase a feeling of vulnerability; involvement in crime; being homeless or living in insecure housing; exposure to drug use within the family; and family break-up. The Royal College of Psychiatrists (1999c) advises that the reasons that lead to drug misuse relate to the effects of the drugs themselves. Taking drugs makes you feel better, at least for a while, which leads individuals (particularly those who are unhappy, stressed or lonely) to keep taking drugs to forget their problems. A pattern can then develop: instead of the individual controlling their own use of the drug, the drug seems to be controlling them.

According to Mind Out For Mental Health (http://mindout.clarity.uk.net/iwi/iP2-addictions.asp, accessed February 2005), there are two levels of addiction: physical and psychological. 'Most people experience both, but they vary according to how long and how much a substance people have been using... But psychological addiction — or "craving" — is harder to overcome, and people can experience anxiety, depression, disrupted sleep and poor concentration, which can make it harder to cope with daily life.'

The Royal College of Psychiatrists (2004a) lists several signs that children or young people may have developed a habit or addiction: unexplained moodiness; behaviour that is 'out of character'; loss of interest in school or friends; unexplained loss of clothes or money; unusual smells; and silver foil. Four questions — to which a 'yes' answer may also indicate that an individual has developed a habit — are:

1. Do you think about drugs every day?
2. Can you say 'no' when they are offered?
3. Would you drink/take drugs alone?
4. Does taking drugs get in the way of the rest of your life?

Source: Royal College of Psychiatrists (2004b)

The Government set out their ten-year strategy for tackling drug misuse in 1998 with a target of reducing the proportion of people under the age of twenty-five reporting the use of Class A drugs by 25% by 2005 and by 50% by 2008 (DoH, 1998a). Boys *et al* (2001) advocate that prevention efforts should be targeted at the general motivations behind taking drugs, as opposed to targeting specific drugs in isolation.

Suicide

Suicide is the second most common cause of death in males in the age group fifteen to thirty-four.

McQueen and Henwood (2002)

WHO estimates that about one million people kill themselves every year — a toll comparable to that of malaria. Worse, on present tends, WHO expects the number to climb to about 1.5 million by 2030.

Brown (2001)

In the year 2000, approximately one million people die by suicide and between ten and twenty times that number attempted suicide. At least five or six people are affected by an individual's suicidal behaviour and therefore at least one hundred million people worldwide have direct contact with suicidal behaviour each year.

Goldney (2002)

The rate of suicide in young men in Scotland is much higher than the rate for the UK as a whole (Scottish Executive, 2002a). Stark *et al* (2002) report that, in the Highlands of Scotland, farmers and crofters were the single largest occupational group dying by suicide. Repper (1999) notes that farmers are 1.5–2 times more likely to commit suicide than men in the general population.

The DoH (1999) explains that certain occupational groups are at greater risk because they have easier access to the means by which to commit suicide. They list these groups as doctors, nurses, pharmacists, vets and farmers.

Younger people who commit suicide more often have a history of schizophrenia, personality disorder, drug or alcohol misuse, and violence (Royal College of Psychiatrists, 2002). Brown (2001) notes that psychiatrists have several theories as to why young people commit suicide, which include the rapid changes in employment, and political and economic environments that have left people bereft of ideals and thus a lost sense of the future, which in turn impinges on their ability to cope. A lack of role model in parents or positive role models to emulate is also a theory. Coleman and Hendry (1999) propose that the increase is due to rising unemployment, alcohol and drug abuse, and an increase in the availability of the means by which to commit suicide. They state that after accidents, suicide is the second most common cause of death in the young, but point out that it is rare under age fifteen years.

'Approximately a quarter of those who take their own life have attempted suicide previously and about half have previously consulted a mental health professional. Many adolescents with suicidal behaviour show low self-esteem and a tendency to social withdrawal and isolation' (www.samaritans.org.uk, accessed February 2005). The Royal College of Psychiatrists (2002) provides more specific information in that two out of three people who commit suicide will have seen their GP in the previous four weeks and nearly half have done so in the week before they kill themselves. Two out of three people who commit suicide will have talked about it with a friend or family member. Individuals who have depression are 22–36 times more likely to commit suicide than mentally healthy people (Brown, 2001).

General suicide factors

⌘   Social adversity and isolation is common.
⌘   Seventy-one per cent of those who commit suicide were unmarried.
⌘   Of those over sixty-five years of age, 41% were widowed.
⌘   Most are either unemployed or long-term sick.

Source: Appleby *et al* (2001)

Suicide factors associated with men

⌘   Difficulties relating to how men express emotions and 'show passion'.
⌘   Pressures associated with debt and child support.
⌘   Isolation.

Source: Scottish Executive (2002b)

Box 6.7: Key facts about suicide

⌘ The second most common cause of death among people under the age of thirty-five is suicide.

⌘ More young men commit suicide than die in road traffic accidents.

⌘ 2005 statistics show that suic ide attempts in young men have fallen by 30% from their peak in 1998. However, the suicide rate in young men remains higher than in the rest of the general population.

⌘ The fall in the suicide rate is partially attributed to a reduction in the availability of over-the-counter aspirin and paracetamol, which is part of the National Suicide Prevention Strategy.

⌘ Numbers of suicides have fallen in older adults.

⌘ One in five of all deaths in young people is due to suicide.

⌘ Although the overall rate of suicide is falling, there are more than 4700 suicides in England and Wales each year.

⌘ In Scotland, over 600 people commit suicide every year, which is one of the highest rates in Europe.

⌘ For every one woman who commits suicide in Ireland and the UK, there are four or five men.

⌘ An unskilled man is over five times more likely to commit suicide than his professional counterpart. Rates in partly skilled and manual skilled workers are twice as high as in the professional group.

⌘ Only one in five young adults (sixteen to twenty-four years) with suicidal thoughts seeks help from a GP. Young men are particularly unlikely to do so unless severely distressed and tend not to seek lay support.

⌘ Cultural or regional influences affect the choice of suicide method. For example, farmers are more likely to shoot themselves because they often have access to shotguns.

⌘ The risk factors for suicide in young people are: mental illness; a family history of mental illness and/or suicide; substance misuse disorders; unemployment; being socially isolated and/or unmarried; recent relationship problems.

Sources: DoH (2002); Scottish Executive (2002a); White and Cash (2003); Men's Health Forum Ireland (2004); Samaritans (2004); Boyle *et al* (2005); Mind out for Mental Health (http://mindout.clarity.uk.net/ppail3-facts-print.asp) (accessed February 2005); NIMHE (2005)

Suicide factors associated with people from minority ethnic communities

⌘　Tensions between the values and ways of life of different cultures and different generations.

⌘　Conflicting perspectives on the role of women and on arranged marriages.

⌘　Experiences associated with being a refugee or asylum-seeker.

Source: Scottish Executive (2002b)

Suicide factors in adolescents and young people

⌘　High degree of family problems.

⌘　Parental disharmony.

⌘　Family deprivation and poverty.

⌘　Parental mental illness.

⌘　Physical and sexual abuse of the child or adolescent by parents.

⌘　Victimisation by peers.

⌘　Unemployment.

Sources: Agerbo *et al* (2002); www.samaritans.org.uk
(accessed February 2005)

The Scottish Executive (2002b) adds the following to the list above:

• 　issues of identity (culture, gender, sexuality)

• 　lack of support eg. among isolated young men or young people leaving care

• 　pressures to achieve and succeed (academically, socially, materially).

The Men's Health Forum (2001) did a study to investigate young men and suicide aptly called 'Soldier It.' They found that young men attempted to supress their feelings as there was a strongly held view that showing emotions led to vulnerability and lack of control, which did not equate with their stereotypical view of masculinity. They believed that they should 'soldier it' and cope with their own problems. Common ways of coping used strategies that would help them (albeit temporarily) to forget their problems, such as using drugs, smoking, alcohol, listening to music, and going to the gym or playing sport. Individuals who have attempted suicide but were unsuccessful (parasuicide) have a 100-times higher risk of suicide in the following year compared with the general population (Jenkins *et al*, 2002).

What can be done to help?

Goldney (2002) cites WHO in 1993, which presented six broad approaches to preventing suicidal behaviour:

1. Treatment of those with mental disorders.
2. Gun possession control.
3. Detoxification of domestic gas (this correlated with reductions in suicide rates in the UK, Japan and Switzerland).
4. Detoxification of car emissions (this correlated with reductions in suicide rates in, again, the UK, Japan and Switzerland).
5. Toning down of reports of suicide in the press (with the aim of reducing rates of those imitating others).
6. Control of availability of toxic substances.

There are a variety of strategies in place to reduce rates of depression and suicide. Mental health is one of the four target areas in *Saving Lives: Our Healthier Nation*. There is a specific target set to reduce suicide by one fifth by 2010. Standard 7 in the *National Service Framework for Mental Health* focuses on preventing suicide. This standard can be seen in *Box 6.8* (overleaf).

In Scotland, the 'Choose Life' National Strategy and Action Plan (2002a) aims to reduce the rate of suicide by 20% by 2013. It has seven objectives:

1. Early prevention and intervention — by providing earlier intervention and support to prevent problems and reduce the risks that might lead to suicidal behaviour.
2. Responding to immediate crisis — by providing support and services to people at risk/in crisis; to provide an immediate response; and to help reduce the severity of any immediate problem.
3. Longer-term work to provide hope and support recovery — providing on-going support and service to enable people to recover and deal with the issues that may be contributing to their suicidal behaviour.
4. Coping with suicidal behaviour and suicide — providing effective support to those who are affected by suicidal behaviour or a suicide.
5. Promoting greater public awareness and encouraging people to seek help early — ensuring greater public awareness of positive mental health and well-being, suicidal behaviour, potential problems and risks amongst all age groups and encouraging people to seek help early.
6. Supporting the media — ensuring that any depiction or reporting by all sections of the media of a suicide or suicidal behaviour is done sensitively and appropriately, and with due respect to confidentiality.

7.   Knowing what works — improving the quality, collection, availability and dissemination of information on issues relating to suicidal behaviour (and self-harm) and on effective interventions to ensure the better design and implementation of responses, services and use of resources.

Box 6.8: Standard 7 — preventing suicide

Local health and social care communities should prevent suicides by:

❀ Promoting mental health for all, working with individuals and communities (Standard One).
❀ Delivering high-quality primary mental health (Standard Two).
❀ Ensuring that anyone with a mental health problem can contact local services via the primary care team, a helpline or an A&E department (Standard Three).
❀ Ensuring that individuals with severe and enduring mental illness have a care plan that meets their specific needs, including access to services round the clock (Standard Four).
❀ Providing safe hospital accommodation for individuals who need it (Standard Five).
❀ Enabling individuals caring for someone with severe mental illness to receive the support they need to continue to care (Standard Six).

And in addition:

❀ Support local prison staff in preventing suicide among prisoners.
❀ Ensure that staff are competent to assess the risk of suicide among individuals at greatest risk.
❀ Develop local systems for suicide audit to learn lessons and take any necessary action.

Source: DoH (1999)

As part of the National Programme in Scotland, a campaign called SeeMe (www.seemescotland.org/) was launched to tackle the stigma that can be associated with mental health problems.

Brown (2001: 1177) points out that more research is now being undertaken into investigating protective factors against becoming suicidal. She states that although such research is still in its infancy 'one striking protective factor seems who dealt with suicides in England and Wales believed that suicide could have been prevented. The associated figures in Northern Ireland and Scotland were 19% and 13%, respectively. The suggested methods to reduce the likelihood of suicide included ensuring better compliance with treatment (especially in young people); closer patient supervision; closer contact with the patient's family; and better staff training.

The Scottish Executive's National Strategy for the prevention of suicide offers some key points in relation to access to help and support:

⌘ Men tend to be reluctant to seek advice and support from health services.

⌘ Young people can be deterred from consulting the family doctor because they are concerned about confidentiality.

⌘ Ethnic-minority communities may not perceive services as acceptable or as culturally competent; language barriers can further impede use.

⌘ Carers report frustration and anger at being turned away and not listened to; confidentiality can block communication.

⌘ Workers in key front-line services (welfare benefits, primary health care, police, residential child care, support workers) lack mental health awareness to be able to support people or to direct them to specialist services.

⌘ Services are not equipped to be able to work effectively with people who are in distress, lead disorganised lives, and find it hard to keep to appointments.

What helps?

In crisis

⌘ Help that is not judgmental.

⌘ Somewhere to feel safe and protected.

⌘ Listening to what those close to the person say.

⌘ Support for families.

⌘ Support for workers.

Preventing problems developing or becoming worse

⌘   A trusting relationship with someone who understands and respects you.

⌘   Coping with and expressing emotions by enabling people to 'give shape to their pain'.

⌘   Help to understand the causes and the triggers that lead to self-harm.

⌘   Persistence, not just short-term support.

⌘   Finding or rebuilding hope of recovery and pleasure in life.

Promoting well-being and capacity to cope

⌘   Developing the emotional literacy of children and young people

⌘   Reviewing the pressures and expectations on young people to achieve

⌘   Actively pursuing social inclusion; valuing diversity, whilst fostering belonging

⌘   Building/protecting social networks and informal supports

Source: Scottish Executive (2002: 3)

Useful websites (all last accessed January 2005)

@ease — an interactive, user-friendly mental health website for young people who are under stress or worried about their thoughts and feelings http://www.rethink.org/at-ease/

Anti-bullying network — a website that offers guidance and information on tackling school bullies — www.antibullying.net

BBC — information on different mental health problems and what to do if someone discusses their feelings of suicide with you — http://www.bbc.co.uk/health/mens/mind_suicide.shtml

BBC Online: Mental Health — accessible, comprehensive information on a wide range of mental health conditions as well as resources for getting help and treatment — www.bbc.co.uk/health/mental

Bully Online — contains information on the prevention of bullying at work and at school — www.successunlimited.co.uk

Calmzone — online home of the Campaign Against Living Miserably. Aimed at raising awareness of depression among young men (especially in Manchester, Merseyside, Cumbria and Bedfordshire) — www.thecalmzone.net

Depression Alliance — www.depressionalliance.org

Effective Interventions Unit — services for young people with problematic drug misue — www.drugmisuse.isdscotland.org/eiu/eiu.htm

Emental-health — a mental health website for doctors and the general public focusing on depression, manic depression, Alzheimer's disease and schizophrenia — www.emental-health.com

FMH — For Mental Health — aims to help young men under twenty-five to take a look at what's going on inside their heads and provide advice, support and information — www.fmhsussex.co.uk

Gamian Europe (Global Alliance of Mental Illness Advocacy Networks) — www.gamian.org/

Health Education Board in Scotland — www.hebs.com/suicideprevention

Hyperguide to the Mental Health Act — www.hyperguide.co.uk/mha

Mentality — a national charity dedicated to the promotion of mental health — www.mentality.org.uk

Mental Health Foundation — leading UK charity providing research and community projects to improve support for people with mental health problems and learning disabilities — www.mentalhealth.org.uk

Mind — leading mental health charity in England and Wales — www.mind.org.uk

NHS Direct Online — www.nhsdirect.nhs.uk

Rethink — working together to help everyone affected by severe mental illness, including schizophrenia, to recover a better quality of life — www.rethink.org/

Royal College of Psychiatrists — professional and educational body for psychiatrists in the UK and Ireland — www.rcpsych.ac.uk

Samaritans — registered charity based in the UK and Ireland for confidential emotional support for people in crisis or at risk of suicide — www.samaritans.org

Sane — charity concerned with improving the lives of everyone affected by mental illness — www.sane.org.uk

Scottish Association for Mental Health — www.samh.org.uk

SPEAR (Self-Preservation Encouraging Active Response) — a support group that runs a correspondence course to help those who self-harm — www.projectspear.com/index1.htm

Survivors UK — helpline and counselling for sexually abused men — www.malesurvivor.org

WHO — statistics on suicide rates across the world — http://www5.who.int/mental_health/main.cfm?p=0000000021

References

Agerbo E, Nordentoft M, Mortensen PB (2002) Familial, psychiatric and socioeconomic risk factors for suicide in young people: nested case-control study. *BMJ* **325**: 74–8

Alexander J (2001) Depressed men: an exploratory study of close relationships. *J Psychiatr Ment Health Nurs* **8**: 67–75

Appleby L, Shaw J, Sherratt J, Amos T, Robinson J, McDonnel R (2001) *Safety First: Five Year Report of the National Confidential Inquiry into Suicide and Homicide by People with Mental Illness*. London: NICE & University of Manchester

Australia's National Mental Health Strategy (2000) *Promotion, Prevention and Early Intervention for Mental Health — A Monograph*. Mental Health Special Programs Branch. Canberra: Commonwealth Department of Health and Aged Care

Bellis MA, Hughes K, Lowey H (2002) Healthy nightclubs and recreational substance use: from a harm minimisation to a healthy settings approach. *Addict Behav* **27**: 1025–35

Bennett DL, Bauman A (2000) Adolescent mental health and risky sexual behaviour. *BMJ* **321**: 251–2

Boreham R, Shaw A (eds) (2001) *Smoking, Drinking and Drug Use Among Young People in England in 2000*. London: HMSO

Boys A, Marsden J, Strang J (2001) Understanding reasons for drug use amongst young people: a functional perspective. *Health Educ Res* **16**(4): 457–69

Braunholz S, Davidson S, King S (2004) *Well? What do you think?* Edinburgh: Scottish Executive Social Research

British Heart Foundation (BHF) (2002) Coronary Heart Disease Statistics. www.bhf.org.uk/professional/index.asp?secID=15&secondlevel=519

British Heart Foundation (2004) Stress and your Heart. http://www.bhf.org.uk/publications/uploaded/bhf_stress.pdf accessed February 2005

Brown P (2001) Choosing to die — a growing epidemic among the young. *Bull World Health Organ* **79**(12): 1175–7

Brunner EM, Marmot M (1999) Social organisational stress and health. In: Marmot, MG, Wilkinson RG (eds) *The Social Determination of Health*. Oxford: OUP

CHI (2003) What CHI has found in mental health trusts: a sector report. http://www.chi.nhs.uk/eng/cgr/mental_health/mental_health_report03.pdf last accessed February 2005

Christie B (2001) Suicide rate in young men in Scotland is twice that in England & Wales. *BMJ* **323**: 888

Coleman JC, Hendry LB (1999) *Adolescent Health*. 3rd ed. London: Routledge

Coulthard M, Farrell M, Singleton N, Meltzer H (2002) *Tobacco, Alcohol and Drug Use and Mental Health*. Norwich: HMSO

Courtenay WH (2000) Constructions of masculinity and their influence on men's well-being: a theory of gender and health. *Soc Sci Med* **50**: 1385–1401

Davidson N, Lloyd T (eds) (2001) *Promoting Men's Health: A Guide for Practitioners*. Edinburgh: Bailliere Tindall

Davies S, Naik PC, Lee AS (2001) Depression, suicide, and the national service framework. *BMJ* **322**: 1500–01

DeVries MW, Wilkerson B (2003) Stress, work and mental health: a global perspective. *Acta Neuropsychaitrica* **15**: 44–53

DoH (1998a) *Tackling Drugs to Build a Better Britain.* London: Stationery Office

DoH (1998b) *Health Survey for England 1996. Volume 1. Findings.* London: Stationery Office

DoH (1999) *Modern Standards and Service Models: A National Service Framework for Mental Health.* London: Stationery Office

DoH (2001a) *Making it Happen: A Guide to Delivering Mental Health Promotion.* London: Stationery Office

DoH (2001b) *Safety First: Five Year Report of the National Confidential Inquiry into Suicide and Homicide by People with Mental Illness.* London: DoH

DoH (2002a) *Summary of the 2002 Cross-Cutting Review.* London: Stationery Office

DoH (2002b) *Tackling Health Inequalities.* London: Stationery Office

DoH (2002c) *National Suicide Prevention Strategy for England.* London: Stationery Office

Elgie R (2002) Mental illness: the need to raise awareness of depression in men. *Men's Health J* **1**(3): 77–9

Ewles L, Simnett I (2003) *Promoting Health: A Practical Guide.* Edinburgh: Bailliere Tindall

Faltermeyer TS and Pryjmachuk S (2000) Men's health: concepts, criticisms and challenges. In: Kerr (ed) *Community Health Promotion: Challenges for Practice.* London: Bailliere Tindall

Faulkner G, Biddle S (1999) Exercise as an adjunct treatment for schizophrenia: a review of the literature. *J Mental Health* **8**(5): 441–57

Faulkner G, Biddle S (2002) Mental health nursing and promotion of physical activity. *J Psychiatr Ment Health Nur* **9**: 659–65

Gelder M (2001) The Royal College of Psychiatrists' survey of public opinion about mentally ill people. http://www.stigma.org/everyfamily/everymain.html

Gilbody S, Whitty P (2002) Improving the recognition and management of depression in primary care. *Eff Health Care* **7**(5): 1–12

Glendinning R, Rose N, Buchanan T, Hallam A (2002) Well? What Do You Think? A National Scottish Survey of Public Attitudes to Mental Health, Well Being and Mental Health Problems. Health and Community Care. Research Findings 27. Edinburgh: Scottish Executive Social Research, www.scotland.gov.uk/socialresearch

Goldney RD (2002) A global view of suicidal behaviour. *Emerg Med* **14**: 24–34

Harrison D (2000) *Understanding Self-Harm.* London: Mind Publications

Hawton K, Rodham K, Evans E, Weatherall R (2002) Deliberate self harm in adolescents: self report survey in schools in England. *BMJ* **325**: 1207–11

Health and Safety Authority (2002) Work-Related Stress Costs EU €20bn a Year. www.hsa.ie/publisher/index.jsp?aID=216&nID=203&pID=201, accessed February 2005

Health and Safety Executive (2000) Work-Related Stress. www.hse.gov.uk/stress/index.htm accessed February 2005

Health and Safety Executive (2004a) *Work-Related Stress*. London: Health and Safety Executive. www.hse.gov.uk/stress/ accessed February 2005

Health and Safety Executive (2004b) *Work-Related Stress*. London: Health and Safety Executive

Hemingway H, Marmot M (1999) Psychological factors in the aetiology and prognosis of coronary heart disease: a systematic review of prospective cohort studies. *BMJ* **318**: 1460–7

Herrman H (2001) The need for mental health promotion. *Aust N Z J Psychiatry* **35**: 709–15

Home Office Drugs Safety Directorate (2002) Updated Drug Strategy 2002. www.drugs.gov.uk/ReportsandPublications/NationalStrategy/1038840683/Updated_Drug_Strategy_2002.pdf accessed February 2005

ICN (2001) World Health Day — 7th April 2001. 'Mental Health: Stop Exclusion Dare to Care.' International Council of Nurses. www.icn.ch/matters_mentalhealth.htm (accessed October 2002)

Jenkins GR, Hale R, Papanastassiou M, Crawford MJ, Tyrer P (2002) Suicide rate 22 years after parasuicide: cohort study. *BMJ* **325**: 1155

Kivimaki M, Leino-Arjas P, Luukkonen R, Riihimaki H, Vahtera J, Kirjonen J (2002) Work stress and risk of cardiovascular mortality: prospective cohort study of industrial employees. *BMJ* **325**: 857–61

Lloyd T, Forrest S (2001) *Boy's and Young Men's Health: Literature and Practice Review*. London: Health Development Agency

Luck M, Bamford M, Williamson P (2000) *Men's Health: Perspectives, Diversity and Paradox*. Oxford: Blackwell Science

Mayor S (2000) Suicide in young men needs multiagency solutions. *BMJ* **320**: 1096

McQueen C, Henwood K (2002) Young men in 'crisis': attending to the language of teenage boy's distress. *Soc Sci Med* **55**: 1493–1509

Men's Health Forum (2001) Young men and suicide: strategy guidelines for health authorities. Men's Health Forum. www.menshealthforum.org.uk/uploaded_files/mhfsuicidestrategy.pdf accessed February 2005

Men's Health Forum (2002) Soldier it! Young men and suicide. Men's Health Forum. www.menshealthforum.org.uk/uploaded_files/mhfsuicideauditfinal.pdf accessed February 2005

Mental Health Foundation (2003) Statistics on Mental Health http://www.mentalhealth.org.uk/page.cfm?pagecode=PMMHST (last accessed February 2005)

National Institute for Mental Health in England (2004a) *Celebrating our Cultures: Guidelines for Mental Health Promotion with the Irish Community*. London: DoH

National Institute of Mental Health in England (2004b) *Celebrating our Cultures: Guidelines for Mental Health Promotion with Black and Minority Ethnic Communities*. London: DoH

NIMHE (2005) *National Suicide Prevention Strategy for England: Annual Report 2004*. Leeds: DoH

ODPM (2004a) *Mental Health and Social Exclusion: Social Exclusion Unit Report.* London: Office of the Deputy Prime Minister Publications

ODPM (2004b) *Action on Mental Health: a Guide to Promoting Social Inclusion.* London: Office of the Deputy Prime Minister Publications

Mulholland C (2000) Depression and suicide in men. www.netdoctor.co.uk/ menshealth/facts/depressionsuicide.htm (accessed April 2003)

Office for National Statistics (2000) *Social Trends 30.* London: Stationery Office

Pollock K, Grime J (2002) Patients' perceptions of entitlement to time in general practice consultations for depression: qualitative study. *BMJ* **325**: 687–92

Prior L, Wood F, Lewis G, Pill R (2003) Stigma revisited, disclosure of emotional problems in primary care consultations in Wales. *Soc Sci Med* **56**: 2191–200

Repper J (1999) A review of the literature on the prevention of suicide through interventions in Accident and Emergency Departments. *J Clin Nurs* **8**: 3–12

Ritchie D (1999) Young mens' perceptions of emotional health: research to practice. *Health Educ* **2**: 70–5

Robertson AE (1998) The mental health experiences of gay men: a research study exploring gay men's health needs. *J Psychiatr Ment Health Nurs* **5**: 33–40

Royal College of Psychiatrists (2002) Men Behaving Sadly. London: Royal College of Psychiatrists www.rcpsych.ac.uk/info/help/mbs/index.htm (accessed February 2005)

Royal College of Psychiatrists (2004a) *Information about Drugs: What Parents Need to Know: Factsheet for Parents and Teachers 30b.* London: Royal College of Psychiatrists

Royal College of Psychiatrists (2004b) *Drugs and Alcohol Factsheet for Young People 36.* London: Royal College of Psychiatrists

Samaritans (2004) Young People and Suicide. www.samaritans.org/know/ informationsheets/youngpeople/young_people_and_suicide_sheet.shtm#overview accessed February 2005

Samaritans with Professor Cary Cooper (2001) Coping with Stress. www.samaritans.org.uk (accessed April 2003)

Scottish Executive (2002a) *Choose Life: A National Strategy & Action Plan to Prevent Suicide in Scotland.* Edinburgh: Scottish Executive

Scottish Executive (2002b) *National Framework for the Prevention of Suicide in Scotland.* Edinburgh: Health Department, Public Health Division, Scottish Executive

Sleath B, Rubin RH (2002) Gender, ethnicity and physician-patient communication about depression and anxiety in primary care. *Patient Educ Couns* **48**: 243–52

Stark C, Matthewson F, O'Neill N, Oates K, Hay A (2002) Suicide in the Highlands of Scotland. Health Bulletin **60**(1): 6–14

Wanless D (2002) *Securing our Future Health: Taking a Long-term View. Final Report.* London: HM Treasury

Warm A, Murray C, Fox L (2003) Why do people self-harm? *Psychol Health Med* **8**(1): 71–9

White A (2001) *Report on the Scoping Study on Men's Health.* London

Wilkerson B (2002) Top 10 Sources of Workplace Stress. www.mentalhealthroundtable.ca (accessed January 2005)

Chapter 7

Maintaining sexual health

Sexually transmitted infections (STIs) are a major cause of ill-health and can have serious consequences, such as infertility.

www.brook.org.uk/content/Fact5_STIs.pdf

You don't need to have a lot of sexual partners to get an STI — almost anyone who is sexually active can get one if you have sex without using condoms.

www.fpa.org.uk/helpnow/sti/

There is a strong link between social deprivation and STIs. The rates of gonorrhoea in some inner-city black and minority ethnic groups, for instance, are ten or eleven times higher than in whites.

www.brook.org.uk/content/M6_2_5_stis.asp

'Sexual health is an essential component of general health and includes the avoidance of unintended pregnancies and sexually transmitted infections' (Nicoll *et al*, 1999: 1321). Another definition: 'sexual health is an important part of physical and mental health. It is a key part of our identity as human beings together with the fundamental human rights to privacy, a family life and living free from discrimination. Essential elements of good sexual health are equitable relationships and sexual fulfilment with access to information and services to avoid the risk of unintended pregnancy, illness or disease' (DoH, 2001a: 5). Perhaps a more basic definition is provided by Flowers *et al* (1999: 484) who cite Greenhouse (1995): 'Sexual health is the enjoyment of sexual activity of one's choice, without causing or suffering physical or mental harm.'

Boys learn from a young age which behaviour is expected of them. It is reported that they often miss out on sex education within the home, whilst sex education within schools is predominantly focused on the biological aspects of reproduction rather than on the impact of masculinity on attitudes and behaviour. So, boys are expected to know about sex and to indulge in sexual practices at an early age. The pressure on young men to live up to the cultural norm and the level of peer pressure to be sexually active and sexually successful is immense. This in turn can lead young men to indulge in risk-taking behaviours in order to prove their manhood (DoH, 2001b).

The average age of first sexual intercourse is seventeen; forty years ago it was twenty-one for women and twenty for men. Lloyd and Forrest (2001: 27) state that it 'is clear that for most young men first heterosexual intercourse takes place between the ages fourteen and seventeen. For the majority, the context is often within a short relationship with a young woman who is known to them, even though not one described as a steady partner. Both young men and women typically describe their chief motivations as curiosity and feeling that intercourse is a natural progression from other sexual contact. However, young men more often report that a desire to lose their virginity motivates them, as does a perception that their male peers are sexually active and their own sexual activity will maintain or enhance their status in this peer group. Alcohol and other drug-use play a part in expediting first intercourse.' A survey of 220 Scots between sixteen and twenty years of age reported that 50% had consumed alcohol at the time of their first sexual encounter, and of these only 13% used a condom compared with 57% of those who had not drunk alcohol (Hooke *et al*, 2000).

It is reported that over 25% of fourteen to fifteen year-olds wrongly believe that the contraceptive pill guards against sexually transmitted infection; that 58% of gay men under twenty years of age do not always wear a condom; and that 44% of HIV-positive men had anal sex with a new partner in the last month, of whom 40% reported no or inconsistent use of condoms (DoH, 2001a).

Wallace and Carlin's (2001) study aimed to identify men's knowledge and attitude to contraception. They used a cross-sectional survey using a questionnaire of 999 men attending a Genito-Urinary Medicine clinic (GUM) which had a 97.2% response rate. The key finding from this study was that 96% of men used contraception with their regular partner to avoid a pregnancy. However, when it came to having intercourse with a casual sex-partner, only 41% of men would always use a condom and 7% stated they never used a condom in this situation. As the authors point out, the latter is worrying since all the respondents were attending a GUM clinic for a sexually transmitted infection (STI).

Nicoll *et al* (1999) reviewed all national routine data pertaining to sexual ill-health among teenagers in England and Wales between the years 1995 and 1996. *Table 7.1* shows the data for men.

Table 7.1: New diagnoses at STI clinics (16–19 year-olds)					
	1995		**1996**		**% rate increase**
	Number	Rate per 1000	Number	Rate per 1000	
Gonorrhoea	687	0.56	895	0.71	31.3
Chlamydia	1197	0.97	1411	1.15	17.9
Genital herpes (first attack)	274	0.22	268	0.22	−2.5
Genital warts (first attack)	1821	1.49	2054	1.68	12.8

These figures, along with those for the female population within the same age group, prompted Nicoll *et al* (1999) to conclude that there is substantial sexual ill-health among teenagers in England and Wales. Sexual ill-health is not equally distributed among the population: the highest burden is borne by women, gay men, teenagers, young adults and black and minority ethnic groups and there is a strong link between social deprivation and STIs, abortions and teenage conceptions (DoH, 2001a). Midgley (2002) adds that Britain is suffering an STI epidemic, especially among young people, She states that in London alone, cases of gonorrhoea have increased by 74% in men and 75% in women since 1995. Syphilis in men has risen by 211% in the past three years and two-thirds of those infections were in heterosexual men.

Chlamydia

GUM [Genito-Urinary Medicine] clinics in England, Wales and Northern Ireland diagnosed 89,818 cases of chlamydia during 2003.

Brook Clinic (2004)

Chlamydia trachomatis infection is the commonest curable STI in the UK. It is very worrying therefore that 40% of young men are unaware that chlamydia is an STI (Brook Clinic, 2004). The highest rates are found in sixteen to nineteen year-old women (791 per 100,000) and in twenty to twenty-four year-old men (465 per 100,000). The incidence of chlamydia is therefore higher in women than in men. Kane *et al* (2001) report a geographical variation in incidence. In 1999, the incidence rates were highest for both men and women in London. Outside London, the highest rates for men were in the north-west and Trent areas in England and lowest in Wales and Northern Ireland. The highest rates for women, outside London, were in Trent, Yorkshire and the north-west area of England, and lowest in Scotland and Northern Ireland. According to the Brook Clinic (2004), chlamydia cases increased by 192% between 1995 and 2003. The incidence is highest in men and women aged twenty to twenty-four.

Since this infection is often asymptomatic (50% of men and 70% of women have no symptoms), control of the infection is more difficult. It often goes undiagnosed, so the true prevalence is unknown. However, it is estimated that it is present in 10% in the under-twenty age-group. In women, the infection can cause damage to the fallopian tubes, causing infertility, and in men it can cause an unusual discharge from the penis; pain when passing urine; pain during sex; testicular pain or swelling (epidyimo-orchitis), which can affect the transport of sperm and have a negative affect on fertility (FPA: www.fpa.org.uk/guide/ infectns/index.htm#3; Kane *et al*, 2001; Thompson *et al*, 2001).

Gonorrhoea

Gonorrhoea is caused by a bacteria called *Neisseria Gonorrhoeae* and is the second most common STI in England, Wales and Northern Ireland. According to the Health Protection Agency, the highest rates are found in London and predominantly urban areas affecting the at-risk groups, including homosexual/ bisexual men and black ethnic minority populations. According to the Brook Clinic (2004), between 1995 and 2003 the rates of gonorrhoea infection increased by 39%, and the rate of genital warts among men is the highest in the UK.

GUM clinics in England, Wales and Northern Ireland diagnosed 70,883 cases of genital warts and 24,309 cases of gonorrhoea (Brook Clinic, 2004). These recent rises in gonorrhoea probably reflect increasing unsafe sexual behaviour, particularly among young people and homosexual men. In Scotland, the rates of gonorrhoea infections in men have increased by 11% since 2000 (HPA, 2004).Gonorrhoea most frequently affects men in the age-group twenty to thirty-four. Black men aged twenty to twenty-four are particularly at risk (Brook Clinic, 2004). Ten percent of men with gonorrhoea have no symptoms, but those who do present with a discharge (watery, yellow or green) from their penis and burning pain when passing urine. Gonorrhoea passed on during oral sex usually causes no symptoms, whilst gonorrhoea passed on through anal sex causes irritation or discharge from the anus (Brook Clinic, 2004).

Those most at risk of gonorrhoea are people with multiple sex partners and those who do not practise safe sex. Therefore, the preventative advice is always to practice safe sex by using a condom correctly and consistently, and seek early advice if infection is suspected.

Human immunodeficiency virus (HIV)

> *By the end of 2003, there were an estimated 53,000 people living with HIV in the UK, of whom 14,300 (27%) were unaware of their infection. The total number of HIV-infected patients seen for care in the UK was 37,079 in 2003. Three-quarters of HIV infections, transmitted through heterosexual intercourse, diagnosed in the UK in 2003 were probably acquired in Africa.*

> HPA (2004a: 10)

HIV is primarily contracted through unprotected vaginal or anal sex or by sharing needles or syringes when injecting drugs (Janssen *et al*, 2001; HPA, 2004a). The DoH (2001) estimates that 30,000 people are living with HIV in the UK and a third of those are undiagnosed. About 400 people die each year. The year 2000 saw the highest increase in HIV infections since the start of the epidemic, and it is noticeable that the most of the newly acquired infections were in heterosexual rather than homosexual men. Of the infections diagnosed in heterosexual men, 75% were thought to be acquired abroad.

A 1999 survey of gay men showed that 58% of those under twenty years of age did not always use a condom. Furthermore, 40% of the 44% of men who were HIV-positive had had anal sex with a new partner in the last month and reported no or inconsistent condom usage (DoH, 2001a). There is evidence of an increase in unsafe sex between men since 1996. The proportion of gay men in London reporting unprotected intercourse increased from 32% in 1996 to 44% in 2000 (PHLS, 2002). The target is to reduce by 25% the number of newly acquired HIV infections and gonorrhoea infections by the end of 2007 (DoH, 2001a).

Maintaining sexual health

> *Sexual health is an important part of physical and mental health. It is a key part of our identity as human beings together with the fundamental human rights to privacy, a family life and living free from discrimination. Essential elements of good sexual health are equitable relationships and sexual fulfilment with access to information and services to avoid the risk of unintended pregnancy, illness or disease.*

> Independent Advisory Group for Sexual Health and HIV (2005: 2)

Box 7.1: Key facts about HIV infections in the UK

- ⌘ In 2002, there were 49,500 adults living with HIV, of whom 22,600 were gay and bisexual men. There was a total of 5,542 new cases of HIV diagnosed, which was almost double that of 1997 and most of the new HIV cases (3,152) were heterosexually acquired.
- ⌘ In Wales in 2004, there were about 900 people diagnosed with HIV infection. Of the 900, just over half were attributed to homosexuals and a third to heterosexuals.
- ⌘ In 2003, there were 6,780 new diagnoses of HIV, contributing to a total of 66,554 since the epidemic began.
- ⌘ Since September 2004, there have been 66,554 diagnoses of HIV.
- ⌘ At the end of September 2004, it was reported that 51% of HIV infections had occurred in men having sex with men; 38% through heterosexual sex; 7% through injecting drug use; and 2% from mother to child.
- ⌘ Since the end of 2004, 57% of all HIV diagnoses have been made in London. There have been 61,292 diagnoses in England; 3,929 in Scotland; 930 in Wales; and 322 in Northern Ireland.
- ⌘ In 2003, 6,780 diagnoses of HIV were made. Among the 5,547 whose ethnicity is known, 33% were white; 57% black-African; 4% black-Caribbean; and 1% Asian.
- ⌘ The cost of managing a patient with HIV is £15,000 per year. The total cost of treatment and care in 2002–2003 was estimated to be £345 million.
- ⌘ In 2000, it was estimated that the average lifetime treatment-cost for an HIV-positive person was between £135,000 and £181,000. The HPA stated in 2004 that each HIV infection prevented saves between £500,000 and £1 million over a lifetime.

Sources: Avert.Org (2005); Chief Medical Officer in Wales (2005); HPA (2004b)

According to Catchpole (2001: 1135) 'sexually transmitted infections can be prevented and controlled through three basic strategies:

1. Reducing the risk of transmission in any sexual encounter (such as condom use);
2. reducing the rate of sexual-partner change;
3. and reducing the period of infectiousness in individuals.'

In 2001, the first National Strategy for Sexual Health and HIV was launched by the Department of Health (DoH, 2001a) with the aim of modernising sexual health and HIV services in order to address the rising prevalence of STIs and HIV:

*We need to foster a culture of positive sexual health by making sure
that everyone gets the information they need — without stigma,
fear or embarrassment — so that they can take informed decisions
to prevent STIs, including HIV, and about services. The strategy
recognises that sexual health is important throughout life, and
that people's needs for information and demands for services vary
according to their age, way of life and sexual orientation.*

DoH (2001a: 12)

In the national strategy for sexual health and HIV there are a number of targets set. These are:

- ⌘ To reduce by 25% the number of newly acquired HIV infections and gonorrhoea infections by the end of 2007.

The target for reducing undiagnosed HIV is:

- ⌘ By the end of 2004, all GUM clinic attendees should be offered an HIV test on their first screening for STIs (and subsequently according to risk) with a view to increasing the uptake of the test to those offered by the end of 2004 and to 60% by the end of 2007.
- ⌘ Reducing by 50% the number of previously undiagnosed HIV-infected people attending GUM clinics who remain unaware of their infection after their visit by the end of 2007.

The targets for increasing the uptake of hepatitis B vaccine are:

- ⌘ By the end of 2003, all homosexual and bisexual men attending GUM clinics should be offered hepatitis B immunisation at their first visit.
- ⌘ Expected uptake of the first dose of the vaccine, in those not previously immunised, to reach 80% by the end of 2004 and 90% by the end of 2006.
- ⌘ Expected uptake of the three doses of vaccine, in those not previously immunised, within one of the recommended regimens to reach 50% by the end of 2004 and 70% by the end of 2006.

In 2002, the Department of Health launched the national Sexual Health and HIV Strategy implementation action plan. This contains twenty-seven points, which provide a framework for the delivery of the strategy and sets out detailed milestones towards the goals of better prevention, better services and better support for people with STIs and HIV. The thrust of the strategy is to normalise sexual health problems and develop an integrated service (involving hospital, community and voluntary sectors) to reduce the current epidemic of STIs, particularly among young people (Bacon and Evans, 2002).

Safe sex

Having safe sex means that you and your partner can enjoy sex and reduce the risk of sexually transmitted infections (including HIV) or unplanned pregnancy.

Public Health Strategy Division (2001)

Box 7.2: Key facts about safe sex

⌘ Safer sex doesn't allow an infected partner's blood, semen or vaginal fluid to get inside the other partner's body.

To have safe sex, remember the following:

⌘ Always use a condom when you have vaginal or anal sex. Get used to putting on a condom. They can be part of your foreplay.
⌘ There's a female condom, available from most chemists, which fits inside the vagina.
⌘ You can enjoy foreplay and sex without penetration, such as kissing, masturbation, stroking or massage.
⌘ Use a condom for oral sex so that you have a barrier between the genital areas and the mouth.
⌘ If you are having anal sex, use a stronger condom and plenty of water-based lubricant.
⌘ If you are using a sex toy such as a dildo or vibrator, put a condom over it. Wash the sex toy between activities and use a new condom each time.

Source: Public Health Strategy Division (2001)

Use of condoms

As discussed previously, young people belong to one of the most at-risk groups for STIs. 'The greatest single risk factor in the transmission of sexually transmitted diseases is the non-use or failure of barrier contraceptives, particularly the male condom' (Lloyd and Forrest, 2001). It is argued that by their very nature, young people do not posess the necessary negotiation skills to ensure the effective and consistent use of condoms (PHLS, 2002).

Lloyd and Forrest (2001) state that the data for young men between thirteen and fifteen at first heterosexual intercourse show that 26% report using a condom and 55% no contraceptive. Condom use rises to 37% among those young people experiencing first intercourse between sixteen and seventeen, and peaks at 42% among eighteen to nineteen year-olds. It could be argued that young men in the thirteen to thirty-five age-group do not use condoms as they have more difficulty in obtaining them than their elder peers who can access machines in pubs and clubs.

It is reported that the use of condoms has increased in the UK, but the increasing numbers of sexual partners negates any advantage seen in condom use (PHLS, 2002). Overall, the proportion of the population who reported two or more partners in the last year did not use condoms consistently since 1990 with current figures of 15.5% of men and 10.1% of women, which suggests that unsafe sex practices are increasing (PHLS, 2002).

Interestingly, Lloyd and Forrest (2001) point out that the use of condoms changes throughout a sexual relationship in that condoms may be used at first, but as the relationship progresses, the couple move towards replacing condoms with the female contraceptive pill. This leads to the realisation that men in heterosexual relationships view condoms as preventing unwanted pregnancy rather than protecting against unwanted pregnancy and STIs. However, Lloyd and Forrest also point out that among the most sexually active young men who report having two or more sexual partners in the last week, there is significantly less likelihood of condom use. These young men may fall into the category of men who perceive themselves to be at low risk of infection.

Lloyd and Forrest (2001: 29) write:

> *Among the factors most likely to have a negative influence on young men are the beliefs that condoms will 'interrupt' sex, be embarrassing to use, and may affect their ability to obtain and maintain an erection... Attitudes to condoms and condom use underpin behavioural intention and predict subsequent condom use — young men who are positive about condoms are more likely to use them than their less confident peers. These attitudes seem to be associated with social background factors. Where more sexist attitudes prevail, and there is less confidence about communicating about sex within families and between young people, condom use*

is less easy for young men. These factors may be more prevalent among young men from lower-class backgrounds and those from particularly strong macho cultures and/or religiously conservative views about sexual matters.

In the Teenage Pregnancy Unit's report on guidance for developing contraception and sexual advice to reach boys and young men, a number of key steps are discussed in order to improve mainstream services and to develop targeted initiatives (DoH, 2001b). Within the guidance, it is strongly recommended that local agencies offer condoms to young men either free of charge or at low cost. Furthermore, to encourage more young men to visit family-planning units, all posters should make it clear that young men are welcome to attend. Lloyd and Forrest (2001) note that male attendance at family planning clinics is very poor and, despite more active promotion for young men to attend, only 6% of the attendees are male. Factors thought to account for this low attendance are that family-planning clinics have traditionally targeted women and are staffed predominantly by women.

The Teenage Pregnancy Unit's guidance document also states that helplines and websites are popular with boys and young men because of their anonymity — the sexwise helpline and associated website, ruthinking (www.ruthinking. co.uk), are the ones most commonly publicised nationally (DoH, 2001b). Again, in the same guidance report, there is a suggestion that more opportunities could be taken with, say, sports teams, as this is a good way of raising awareness of sexual health and a way to increase access to condoms.

In relation to the gay community, Lloyd and Forrest (2001: 30) write:

Among gay men, condom use is related to the prevention of infection with sexually transmitted diseases, particularly HIV. The promotion of condom use for anal intercourse has been active and regarded as a success, partly as a result of considerable mobilisation within gay communities. However, as the larger pool of infection is among gay men, exposure to infection is potentially more frequent.

Barriers to 'safe sex'

- ⌘ Reluctance to discuss openly condom use or even sexual intentions, preferring instead just to 'let things happen'.
- ⌘ Difficulties accessing, carrying and using condoms, accompanied by embarrassment and concerns about decreased sensitivity when using a condom.

Sex and relationship education

Effective sex and relationship education can reduce sexual ill-health among young people (DoH, 2001a). However, sex and relationship education involves more than educating young people in the prevention of STIs and unwanted pregnancies. Thistle and Ray (2004: 44), writing about the role of the school nurse in sex and relationship education, argue that it is an education that is sustained over a lengthy period of time in order to support children as they progress from childhood to puberty and adolescence. The aim is to prepare them for adult life in which they:

- are aware of and enjoy their sexuality
- develop positive values and a moral framework that will guide their decisions, judgements and behaviour
- have the confidence and self-esteem to value themselves and others
- behave responsibly within sexual and personal relationships
- communicate effectively
- have sufficient information and skills to protect themselves and their partner from unintended or unwanted conceptions and sexually transmitted infections, including HIV
- neither exploit nor are exploited
- can access confidential advice and support'

Erectile dysfunction

Erectile dysfunction is a disease that produces significant psychological problems for the men who suffer from it. Leung and Yip (1999) explain that erectile dysfunction is the 'inability to achieve and/or maintain an erection that is sufficient for satisfactory sexual activity. Traditionally, the term impotence was used. However, impotence carries a derogatory sense of lack of power with implications for sexual desire, orgasm or ejaculation.'

Erectile dysfunction is a condition affecting at least one in every ten men. It is estimated that there are therefore about 2.3 million men in the UK suffering from erectile dysfunction. According to the Sexual Dysfunction Association, only about 10% of these men actually receive treatment. In February 2002, a news release from the Men's Health Forum stated that over 85% of men with erectile dysfunction take over six months to summon the courage to seek treatment, and nearly 50% delay for over two years. In a study of 500 American men by Levine and Kloner (2000), 74% of men stated that they had not disclosed their problem to a doctor because of embarrassment. Key features of the condition can be seen in *Box 7.3*.

Box 7.3: Key features of erectile dysfunction

✶ Average age of onset — fifty to sixty years.
✶ Occurs mainly as a result of age-related diseases such as diabetes, atherosclerosis and hypertension.
✶ Smoking is a risk factor.
✶ Can occur after prostate surgery.
✶ About 25% of cases can be attributed to side-effects of medications.
✶ Only 20% of cases are attributed to psychological factors.

Source: Levine and Kloner (2000)
More detailed information is supplied by Delvin and Webber (2002) at www.
netdoctor.co.uk/sex_relationships/facts/ed_partner.htm; www.netdoctor.co.uk/
sex_relationships/facts/ed_partner.htm (accessed February 2005)

Psychological causes

- anxiousness about whether you can 'perform'
- problems in the relationship
- depression
- bereavement
- tiredness
- stress
- 'hang-ups' — for instance, guilt about sex
- unresolved gay feelings

Physical causes

- problems with the chemical mechanism that causes an erection to occur (more common in older men)
- high blood pressure or atherosclerosis (hardening of the arteries)
- diabetes
- smoking (which increases the risk of developing atherosclerosis)
- side-effects of anti-hypertensive drugs and some anti-depressant or ulcer-healing drugs

- side-effects of alcohol and cocaine
- major surgery (eg. prostate surgery or other abdominal operations)

Men with hypertension and who also smoke are twenty-six times more likely to suffer from erectile dysfunction than are non-smokers. It is suggested that this is due to the fact that smoking accelerates the development of atherosclerosis (hardening of the arteries). When blood vessels within the pelvic area are narrowed as a result of atherosclerosis, this can cause a reduction in blood flow to the penis, resulting in erectile problems (www.malehealth.co.uk, accessed February 2005). ASH (2004b: 1) report that 'smoking increases the risk of impotence by around 50% for men in their thirties and forties. ASH and the British Medical association have calculated that around 120,000 UK men in this age group are needlessly impotent as a result of smoking.' A list of good questions to check for erectile dysfunction is at www.bbc.co.uk/health/sex/comprobs_impotence.shtml (accessed February 2005).

Specific lifestyle changes such as stopping smoking, losing excess weight, exercising more, and reducing anxiety and stress are suggested measures to adopt in the first instance. However, if symptoms persist then medical advice should be sought from a GP. If that poses difficulty, advice can be obtained from family-planning clinics or GUM clinics (see Sexual Dysfunction Association www.sda.uk.net accessed January 2005).

Useful websites (all last accessed January 2005)

Brook Advisory Centres — www.brook.org.uk

Department for Education and Skills — their sex and relationships education guidance can be downloaded from www.dfes.gov.uk/sreguidance

Family Planning Association — www.fpa.org.uk

Institute of Psychosexual Medicine — www.ipm.org.uk

Men's Health Forum is a charitable organisation that works to improve men's health by bringing together and working with the widest possible range of interested organisations and individuals — www.menshealthforum.org.uk

Sex Education Forum has the latest resources on sex and relationships education and guidance in England — www.ncb.org.uk/sef/

Teenage Pregnancy Unit — www.teenagepregnancyunit.gov.uk

Wired for Health, the national healthy schools website — www.wiredforhealth.gov.uk

Facts on sexually transmitted infections — www.bbc.co.uk/health/mens/cond_stds.shtml

References

Avert.org (2005) UK HIV/AIDs FAQs. www.avert.org/aidsfaqs.htm#q1 (accessed February 2005)

Bacon LE, Evans J (2002) Sexual health services need wider approach. *BMJ* **325**: 1302

Carne C (1998) Sexually transmitted infections. *BMJ* **317**: 129–32

Catchpole M (2001) Sexually transmitted infections: control strategies. *BMJ* **322**: 1135–6

Chief Medical Officer (2005) Health Status Wales 2004–05. Cardiff: Office of the Chief Medical Officer, Welsh Assembly Government

DoH (2001a) *The National Strategy for Sexual Health and HIV*. London: DoH

DoH (2001b) *Guidance for Developing Contraception and Sexual Advice Services to Reach Boys and Young Men*. Teenage Pregnancy Unit, London: DoH

DoH (2002) *National Sexual Health and HIV Strategy Implementation Action Plan*. London: DoH

Flowers P, Hart G, Marriott C (1999) Constructing sexual health. *J Health Psychol* **4**(4): 483–95

Greenhouse P (1995) A definition of sexual health. *BMJ* **310**: 8–9

Independent Advisory Group for Sexual Health and HIV (2005) *Independent Advisory Group for Sexual Health and HIV Annual Report 2003/4*. London: DoH

Hooke A, Capewell S, Whyte M (2000) Gender differences in Aryshire teenagers' attitudes to sexual relationships, responsibility and unintended pregnancies. *J Adolesc* **23**: 477–86

HPA (2004a) *Focus on Prevention: HIV and other Sexually Transmitted Infections in the United Kingdom in 2003. An update November 2004*. London: Health Protection Agency Centre for Infections

HPA (2004b) *Sexually Transmitted Infections. Annual Report & Accounts 2004*. London: Health Protection Agency Centre for Infections

Janssen M, de Wit J, Hospers HJ, van Griensven F (2001) Educational status and young Dutch gay men's beliefs about using condoms. *AIDS Care* **13**(1): 41–56

Kane R, Khadduri R, Wellings K (2001) Screening for chlamydia among adolescents in the UK: a review of policy and practice. *Health Educ* **101**(3): 108–115

Leung LS, Yip AWC (1999) Sildenafil (Viagra) and erectile dysfunction. *Ann Coll Surg* **4**: 99–102

Levine LA, Kloner RA (2000) Importance of asking questions about erectile dysfunction. *Am J Cardiol* **86**: 1210–13

Lloyd T, Forrest S (2001) *Boy's and Young Men's Health; Literature and Practice Review*. London: Health Development Agency

Midgley C (2002) The price of causal sex. *The Times* January 29th

Nicoll A, Catchpole M, Cliffe S, Hughes G, Simms I, Thomas D (1999) Sexual health of teenagers in England & Wales: analysis of national data. *BMJ* **318**: 1321–2

PHLS (2002) Sexual Health in Britain: Recent Changes in High-Risk Sexual Behaviours and Epidemiology of Sexually Transmitted Infections Including HIV. www.phls.org.uk, accessed February 2005

Public Health Strategy Division (2001) Sexual Health for Men. www.hpw.wales.gov. uk, accessed April 2003

Thistle S, Ray C (2002) Sex and relationships education: the role of the school nurse *Nurs Stand* **18**(17): 44–55

Thompson C, Macdonald M, Sutherland S (2001) A family cluster of chlamydia trachomatis infection. *BMJ* **322**: 1473–4

Wallace SVF, Carlin EM (2001) Contraception and men attending a genitourinary medicine clinic. *J Fam Plann Reprod Health Care* **27**(4): 217–20

Chapter 8

Conclusion

Most of the leading causes of death among men are the result of
men's behaviours — gendered behaviours that leave men vulnerable.

Kimmel and Messner (1995)

A sobering message from Frankish (2003) is that unless action is taken now
to address unhealthy lifestyles and reduce smoking rates, the cancer rates
worldwide will rise by 50% over the next twenty years. She refers to the World
Cancer Report (WHO, 2003), which states that the following three areas of
action can reduce the estimated increase in cancer rates by a third:

- ⌘ 'Reduction of tobacco consumption. It remains the most important
  avoidable cancer risk. In the twentieth century, approximately 100
  million people died worldwide from tobacco-associated disease.
- ⌘ A healthy lifestyle and diet can help. Frequent consumption of fruit
  and vegetables and physical activity can make a difference.
- ⌘ Early detection through screening, particularly for cervical and breast
  cancers, allows for prevention and successful cure.'

The website, malehealth, provides men with an analogy of imagining their body
to be a car. This is used in an attempt to normalise health problems that may
occur in men and to suggest that it is equally normal for men to seek help to
rectify the problem — just as they would seek help from a garage for problems
with their car.

Early warning signs — tradesman's tips

'Few men would continue driving with steam pouring out of the radiator or
loose steering, yet we will carry on putting up with many symptoms of early
disease much longer than do women. Here are some early warning signs from
our expert man-mechanics that should not be ignored or you might just find
yourself looking for some pretty vital second-hand parts:

a) **Oil pressure warning light**: high blood pressure has few warning signs. This is why it is called "the silent killer". Check your blood pressure at least once a year before you develop blood in your urine, tunnel vision or have a stroke.

b) **Ignition warning light**: if you are not charging your battery, you will soon not be able to start your engine. Losing weight, a loss of appetite or difficulty in eating needs your doctor's attention.

c) **Rev counter**: if you are over-revving on slight inclines, your engine will wear out prematurely. Being unfit is one cause of a high heart rate, which refuses to return to normal quickly after exercise.

d) **Speedometer**: KPH or MPH, if you can't seem to get past idling speed, you need to see your doctor or think seriously about some more exercise.

e) **Brake warning light**: not being able to resist one more drink with days off work, poor sleep, bad temper and friction at home is a sign of the brakes needing attention.

f) **Main beam warning light**: are you peering into the gloom? Maybe your eyes need testing? Diabetes is a common cause of eye problems.

g) **Temperature gauge**: over-heating is a common sign of obesity. You may find your radiator boiling over as well. This can affect your heart, pancreas and blood vessels, not to mention your erectile function.

h) **Fuel gauge**: trouble with your erections? You may have an underlying condition causing erectile dysfunction or impotence.

i) **Seat belt warning noise**: taking unnecessary risks? Young men are much more likely than older men to risk their lives through driving fast, not wearing protective clothing, and failing to see their doctor when they find something wrong.

j) **Low tyre pressure**: feeling down? Depression is grossly under-diagnosed in men, while suicide is four times higher than in women. Look out for loss of interest, a 'short fuse', alcohol abuse, loss of libido, or thoughts of harming yourself.

k) **High exhaust gas emissions and backfire**: inefficient fuel combustion is similar to poor digestion, which can result from various problems, not least cancer. Blood in your stool is a warning sign not to be ignored.

l) **Engine misfire**: timing is just as important to the heart as it is to the car engine. An irregular heart rate, especially with exercise, needs attention.

m) **Engine labouring**: pain in the chest could be a sign of problems with your heart.

n) **Direction indicator failure**: bad earth? Poor circulation and nerve disorders can cause problems with the body's 'electrics'.

o) **STOP warning indicator**: hopefully, after reading this section, you will never see this indicator come on, or at least not until you can be classified as a vintage model.

Make no mistake, you are in control of your body, but good drivers take heed of warning signs.'

Source: Malehealth website: www.malehealth.co.uk/userpage1.cfm?item_id=548 (accessed January 2005)

It should be apparent after reading this book that to improve men's health, a different approach must be taken to that for women. Men have different health needs and require health services that are tailored to these needs — for example, evening, weekend and drop-in surgeries. Health services need to be more proactive, and to go to men instead of expecting men to come to them. Providing access to health care at work, sporting venues, pubs and community organisations seems to be key (Baker, 2001). Courtenay *et al* (2002) write:

The attitudes and beliefs that one adopts can also have powerful influence on both one's health and one's health behaviour. Men and adolescent males who adopt traditional or stereotypical beliefs about masculinity have greater health risks than their peers with less traditional beliefs. If men are to live longer, healthier lives, they will need to change their unhealthy beliefs and behaviours.

References

Alcohol Concern: www.alcoholconcern.org.uk/publications (accessed April 2003)

Baker P (2001) The state of men's health. *Men's Health J* **1**(1): 6–7

Courtenay WH, McCreary DR, Merighi JR (2002) Gender and ethnic differences in health beliefs and behaviours. *J Health Psychol* **7**(3): 219–31

Frankish H (2003) 15 million new cancer cases per year by 2020, says WHO. *Lancet* **361**: 9365. www.thelancet.com/journal/vol361/iss9365/artid/25286 (accessed April 2003)

Kimmel MS, Messner MA (1995) *Men's Lives*. 3rd ed. Needdham Heights, Mass: Simon & Schuster, cited in Alcohol and Men Factsheet. www.alcoholconcern.org.uk/publications (accessed April 2003)

WHO (2003) World Cancer Report. www.who.int (accessed April 2003)

Index

A

alcohol 6, 8, 9, 10, 11, 12, 23, 28, 34, 35, 36, 43, 44, 45, 47, 52, 53, 77, 78, 79, 80, 81, 82, 84, 85, 86, 87, 124, 128, 129, 130, 132, 134, 136, 139, 144, 146, 157, 168, 172

aspirin 57, 75, 145

B

Bangladeshi men 16, 19, 27, 33, 34, 105

binge drinking 34, 47, 77, 81, 83, 87

Body mass index (BMI) 33, 91

C

chlamydia 158, 159, 169, 170

colorectal cancer 6, 41, 58, 59, 60, 61, 62, 73, 76

condoms 156, 157, 164, 165, 169

coronary heart disease 5, 15, 17, 34, 38, 39, 40, 41, 82, 90, 97, 116, 118, 138, 154

D

depression 7, 16, 34, 91, 93, 117, 122, 128, 129, 130–138, 142, 144, 147, 150–155, 167

diabetes 15, 17, 19, 22, 32–34, 38, 88, 90–97, 104, 106, 107, 113, 114, 115, 118, 122, 167

drug misuse 138, 142, 143

E

emotional problems 7, 155

erectile dysfunction 75, 166, 168, 169, 172

G

gonorrhoea 156, 158, 159, 160, 162

H

heart attack 4, 15, 17, 22, 24, 29, 30, 39, 55, 94, 106, 122

heart disease ii, 1, 5, 15, 17, 23, 32, 34, 37, 38, 39, 40, 41, 50, 51, 54, 81, 82, 90, 96, 97, 100, 106, 116, 118, 131, 138, 154

high blood pressure 1, 15, 22, 122, 167, 172

HIV 6, 24, 140, 142, 157, 160, 161, 162, 163, 165, 166, 169, 170

I

Irish men ii, 27, 35, 41

L

life expectancy 1, ii, 15, 35, 55, 88, 91, 94, 97, 98

lung cancer 24, 29, 30, 41, 44, 46, 47, 48–58, 63, 74, 75, 76

M

masculinity 2, 3, 9, 13, 146, 152, 156, 173

mental health 7, 86, 106, 117–140, 144, 145, 148–156, 160–161

monosaturated fats 100

O

obesity 16, 17, 22, 32, 33, 82, 88–98,
101, 103, 104, 107, 114–116, 172

P

passive smoking 32, 38, 50, 51, 55
physical activity 16, 19, 22, 38, 61, 73,
88, 96, 97, 104–111, 114–116, 137,
153, 171
polyunsaturated fats 99
prostate cancer 1, 32, 41, 42, 58, 62–65,
70–76, 94, 116

R

risk-taking 3, 9, 11, 13, 14, 156
road-traffic accidents 78, 82

S

safe sex 159, 163, 165
saturated fats 19, 47, 88, 100, 101
self-harm 137–139, 148, 150, 151, 155
smoking cessation 31, 36, 53–57, 73, 76
social network 8

socioeconomic factors 16, 27, 36, 81
South Asian men 22, 81, 93
stress 7, 31, 34, 38, 47, 70, 78, 82, 94,
106, 107, 109, 118, 119, 122–128,
138, 150, 152, 154, 167, 168
stroke ii, 15, 17, 22, 29, 32, 35, 36, 51,
55, 82, 88, 93, 96, 97, 106, 107,
118, 122, 136, 172
suicide ii, 24, 118, 129, 133, 138,
143–155, 172

T

testicular cancer ii, 42, 65–68, 72, 73,
74, 75
trans-fats 99, 101

U

unemployment 8, 121, 136, 144, 145,
146

W

work-related stress 34, 70, 123, 124, 128